Controlling Type 2 Diabetes

A Natural Alternative

Elizabeth V Gemmell

NOTES FOR UK READERS

BLOOD GLUCOSE NUMBERS

To convert US to UK divide by 18
To convert UK to US multiply by 18

DATES:

All in the US standard of month, day, year.

"I thoroughly enjoyed reading this book. It is one of the most thorough outlines of Life Style Modifications to control or to prevent Type 2 Diabetes Mellitus. . . . It gives excellent advice to anyone who is dedicated to the first line of treatment of Type 2 Diabetes Mellitus and sends a clear message to patients that drug therapy is an add-on when lifestyle does not offer complete control."

—James W. Reed, MD, MACP, FACE
Professor of Medicine, Associate Chair of Medicine for Research, Chief of Endocrinology, Chief of Medicine Service at Grady for Morehouse School of Medicine, Faculty of The Educational Council of the National Diabetes Educational Initiative, Author of *Living with Diabetes: A Guide to Patients and Parents*

~ ~ ~

". . .an inspiring and empowering story for anyone who is struggling with chronic disease . . . diabetes, high blood pressure, high cholesterol and obesity." . . .who wish to forego a lifetime commitment to drugs and reclaim a healthy lifestyle."

—Audra Hanley, MD

Controlling Type 2 Diabetes

A Natural Alternative

Elizabeth Villiers Gemmette

Please Note

This book is not to be used as a substitute for professional medical advice, diagnosis or treatment. Always consult a physician or other qualified health care professionals with any questions you may have regarding a medical condition or before making any decisions pertaining to illness, health, diet and wellness.

Dedicated to the memory of my husband,
Gerard R. Gemmette,
who died on October 25, 2006

Within a few weeks of my husband's death,
I came across the following note:

HALF MOON HOTEL,
MONTEGO BAY, JAMAICA, WI

July 9, 1976

Elizabeth—

Happy fifth anniversary. I love you very
much and our son is absolutely precious.

May we have another thirty years like this.

Love,
Gerard R.

It is a painful thing
To look at your own trouble and know
That you yourself and no one else has made it.
SOPHOCLES

Table of Contents

Foreword ix

Introduction 1

Part I
One More Diagnosed Diabetic

<u>Chapter</u>
1   Symptoms 6
2   Diagnosis 11
3   Reactions to the Diagnosis 17

Part II
Diabetes Education

4   What Is Diabetes? 24
5   Complications 31
6   Diet and Exercise 36

Part III
More About Diet

7   Fruit, Milk, Protein, and Starches 42
8   Vegetables, Fats, and Alcohol 48
9   Diet Products, Sugar Substitutes, and Sugar 53

Part IV
Reaping the Rewards
10 Positive Progress 58
11 A Full Vasovagal, Without Cream Cheese 63
12 The Moment of Truth 68

Part V
Dealing with Stress
13 Stress Test 76
14 Staying with the Program 81
15 "It's All About Me" 85

Part VI
Refining the Eating Plan
16 Potatoes, Anyone? 92
17 More Starch Experiments 97
18 Weights and Measures 101

Part VII
The What, When and Where of the Diet
19 The Basic Modified Daily Diet 106
20 Breakfast, Lunch, and Dinner 108
21 Eating Out and Fast Food 111

Part VIII
Shopping and Cooking
22 Shopping List/Serving Sizes 116
23 Product Preferences .122
24 Recipes 124

Afterword 149

Foreword

Audra Hanley, M.D.

This is an inspiring and empowering story for anyone who is struggling with chronic disease, more specifically diabetes, high blood pressure, high cholesterol, and obesity.

I am Ms. Gemmette's family practitioner. I rarely meet patients who have the motivation, desire and tenacity to make significant changes in their lives. When Ms. Gemmette insisted that she would manage her diabetes, high blood pressure and cholesterol with diet and exercise, I was compelled to warn her of the significant risk she was taking, particularly given the severity of her conditions. I was skeptical and wondered if I was shirking some paternalistic duty by not being more insistent that she consider pharmaceuticals. Months later when Ms. Gemmette had shed pounds, normalized her blood sugar, blood pressure and cholesterol, I was truly amazed at her progress. I had to reconsider my stance.

Perhaps Western medicine reaches too quickly for pharmaceuticals, and perhaps patients have become too complacent and accept them too willingly. After all, isn't it easier to "pop a pill" than to make a significant change in lifestyle? We know only too well that we must take heed of the side effects of medication and the cost of that medication to our medical system. We are constantly battling rising insurance premiums due to the expense of prescribed pharmaceuticals and the necessity of monitoring them with frequent doctor and lab visits.

Certainly there are cases where pharmaceuticals are unavoidable and critical to appropriate care, but where such use can be avoided by the efforts of the patient, this is the preferred choice of treatment. Perhaps the real message here is that health care is a shared responsibility between the doctor and the patient and that each can learn from the other as we struggle to treat, cure, or manage, a disease.

The author's narrative style is easily accessible to anyone, regardless of medical background. The information is timely with the rise in diabetes and obesity among American adults and makes a bold statement in favor of those patients who wish to forego a lifetime commitment to drugs and reclaim a healthy lifestyle.

INTRODUCTION

The ability to simplify means to eliminate the
unnecessary so that the necessary may speak.
HANS HOFMANN

    This is not a how-to-book. It is meant to be inspirational and motivational. Simply put, this is the story of my decision to try to control type 2 diabetes with diet, exercise and weight loss without the aid of oral drugs. This decision was made with my doctor's knowledge, if not her approval. It is not suggested that the reader follow the same path unless it is approved of by their own doctor and with their own doctor's guidance. People have asked me if I would have taken drugs if my first line of defense had not worked. Well, of course I would. But even if I had had to resort to oral medicine at first and/or insulin later, I still would have followed my own diet, exercise, and weight loss program. There was more than diabetes at stake. My goal was to control type 2 diabetes, rework cholesterol levels, regulate blood pressure and reduce weight in order to reach a new level of health. The results speak for themselves. The reader will note that I have talked about "controlling" type 2 diabetes. Many experts believe that once a person is diabetic, they are always diabetic. The implication is that type 2 diabetes cannot be reversed only controlled. The question becomes: If a person's blood glucose numbers are consistently in the non-diabetic range, is the person still dia-

betic? Although I could articulate some theories of my own on
the topic, I will leave the medical experts to argue over reversing vs. controlling type 2 diabetes. For my part, I believe that
I have controlled a condition caused by my own bad habits.

At the end of this book, I have included some recipes to
show how I have modified a few of my favorite dishes to fit
into my new eating plan and because so many people have
asked me how I lost weight and controlled type 2 diabetes.
The most asked question is "What do you eat?" The other
question I hear a lot is "How difficult was it?" I tell them it was
not difficult at all. All I needed to do was **KEEP IT SIMPLE**.

KNOWLEDGE

EXERCISE

EAT WELL

PORTION CONTROL

INVEST

TEST

SUGAR

I CAN DO THIS

MANAGE STRESS

PROGRAM YOUR HEAD

LOWER THE NUMBERS

ENJOY LIFE

KNOWLEDGE. Knowledge is the key to embarking on a path to
successfully controlling type 2 diabetes. Obtaining the necessary knowledge was easy for me. I simply took my doctor's
advice and attended and participated in the diabetes education
program offered at a local hospital. The professionals involved
in that program provided the basic information about what
causes diabetes, covered the complications of uncontrolled
blood glucose, and offered ways to help to control diabetes and
avoid the complications. There was no need for me to read lots
of medical articles and books. I bought one book on "reversing" diabetes as a reference guide.

EXERCISE. Exercise was already in my schedule. That exercise was quickly upped to 30 minutes a day on the stationary bike, five leg machines, one stomach exercise on the ball, and weights for the arms. Nothing strenuous here.

EAT WELL. One hour with the dietician in the diabetes program was invaluable. After learning what needed to be eliminated from my diet, I engaged in a thorough purging of forbidden foods from the refrigerator and kitchen cabinets. Grocery store shelves were scoured for the right foods. The main goal was to eat only healthy foods.

PORTION CONTROL. Healthy food is not healthy if eaten in unhealthy portions. Learning portion control was critical. The meal planning guide provided in the diabetic classes at the local hospital and published by the American Diabetic Association was particularly useful for understanding portion sizes. It was time to weigh foods and measure drinks. Just a scale, measuring spoons, and measuring cups were all that was needed.

INVEST. Investing in two books on the Glycemic Index helped to refine the diet by determining which foods raise blood glu-cose rapidly and which foods are slow-acting. One book at first, another added much later. Two books were all that was needed.

TEST. From the day of diagnosis, blood glucose testing was done as directed by the doctor. Testing was done as often as recommended and only as often as recommended. There were suggestions from other professionals that blood glucose should be tested before exercise, after exercise, before bed, after certain foods. How easily a compulsion could develop.

SUGAR. Making a decision about sugar and sugar substitutes was easy. There is no room for sugar or for sugar substitutes in my diet. Why? I am not willing to take the chance of developing a sweet tooth. I am not willing to sacrifice good calories for empty calories contained in sugar. I am not willing to risk side effects from the sweeteners.

I CAN DO THIS. This was my mantra as I followed my journey to health. I can do this. Introducing positive thinking into the new program and learning to be patient waiting for positive results was the key to my success.

MANAGE STRESS This might be the hardest mandate in the management of type 2 diabetes. Identifying the causes of stress is a good place to start. After that, there is a searching for ways to relieve that stress. The problem is that worrying about stress is stressful in and of itself. For me, that one hour a day in the gym was as good as it gets.

PROGRAM YOUR HEAD. The head needs to take over from the mouth. I knew that this had taken place when I was unable to swallow a food that I had planned to eat before testing the blood glucose. By all accounts, this was a fairly safe food on the Glycemic Index. I put it in my mouth, but I just couldn't swallow it. That was when I knew candy bars had no chance.

LOWER THE NUMBERS. That's right, the numbers. My goal was not just to lower the Hemoglobin A1c. I needed to lower the bad cholesterol, the blood pressure and the weight. Sneak preview: I lowered my Hemoglobin A1c from 12.9 to 5.7 in just over six months.

ENJOY LIFE. Now that the numbers have been turned around, it's time for the rewards. Not with food. Perhaps with a new wardrobe. After all, there is nothing in my closet that fits anymore. Or perhaps with a trip on a plane, now that I can fit comfortably in the seat.

Part I

One More Diagnosed Diabetic

~ 1 ~

SYMPTOMS

Life is one long process of getting tired.
SAMUEL BUTLER

In January of 2005, my husband and I drove over to Albany to inspect seventy boxes of legal files and pull out pre-nuptial agreements and post-nuptial agreements, or any other important documents, before confirming that the contents of the boxes could be disposed of by the storage company. We were working on destroying more vestiges of a long-established, but now closed, law practice.

The minute we arrived at the dusty old warehouse where records of patients, clients and customers of hospitals, doctors, lawyers, CPA's and many other professionals and businesses are stored in thousands of file boxes, I had this raging thirst. It never occurred to me to ask for a paper cup and drink water from the dirty bathroom faucet. I hadn't drunk tap water since 1979 when I had had a medical scare. Back then, I used to take empty containers to the Spa at Saratoga Springs and fill the bottles with spa water. The medical scare came during my first week of law school. A local cardiologist had said that I had a very serious heart arrhythmia and would surely die if I didn't take the prescribed pills.

With a death scare over my head, I dropped out of law

school and took the prescribed pills. The pills were followed by hallucinations, hair loss, missed periods, and gall bladder attacks—without a gall bladder. After five months, I stopped taking the medicine. During that five months, I had visited the local health food store. We had been on vacation in Bermuda and one person had mentioned that his secretary had cured a similar condition with diet and exercise. Another person mentioned that he knew someone who had good results with a similar condition by visiting a naturopath.

As I roamed the health food store looking for tofu and organic products, I started chatting with the woman behind the counter. She said that there was a naturopathic doctor in Albany who might be able to help me. She would give me his number. The naturopath turned out to be what I needed, although I wasn't sure what I was supposed to do with the vegetarian diet. We soon adapt in times of need. I became a vegetarian and often mixed in health food stores and cafés with young women who wore long skirts and had long flowing untended locks. It was, after all, at the end of the seventies. For me to go somewhat counterculture was a little shocking.

From 1979 until 1998, I had the discipline not to eat meat. During those years, on only three occasions did I put a piece of meat in my mouth—bacon, corned beef and black pudding (pig's blood congealed in pearl barley). Each time, I spat the meat out. Most nights I made a vegetarian meal for myself and a meal centered around meat for my family. It wasn't until 1998 that I faltered. I had made a leg of lamb studded with garlic for the family and the urge to eat meat overcame me. After all, I reasoned, the old heart condition had been taken care of a long time ago. And how many years would I live anyway? No longer a vegetarian. Still not drinking tap water. And very resistant to drugs, even pill phobic.

Now, we were in a warehouse on a back road away from convenience stores and supermarkets and I had this raging unquenchable thirst upon me. I decided then that I would

never leave home again without a bottle of water in my pos-
session. The young woman who was studiously entering file
box numbers into the computer offered to make coffee and I
gulped down a couple of cups with milk and sugar.

After that first episode of being beside myself with
thirst, the problem progressed to the point where I moved
around my house and office only if I had a container with at
least sixteen ounces of water in it with me at all times. I
remember waking one night with such an overpowering thirst
that I went downstairs to the kitchen and drank three sixteen
ounce glasses of water one after the other. Even after that my
mouth felt as though it was stuffed with cotton balls. It was
like the feeling I had after waking up after operations—a C-
Section followed by a gall bladder removal that same year.
Cotton mouth would be the best way to describe it. No matter
how much you beg, the nurse only lets you have a lemon stick
to wipe around your mouth.

You know how we do reality checks when something
seems different or wrong. I kept asking my husband if he ever
got really thirsty. He replied that of course he did and when
that happened the only thing that helped was a soda. Ah,
soda. By March, I was having a soda in the afternoon. I was
drinking big glasses of "healthy" juice. I had become a juicea-
holic. The new juicer sat gleaming on the kitchen counter, and
I enjoyed putting in about seven or eight pieces of fruit, then
pouring the extracted juice into two glasses—one for me and
one for my husband. Then there was the low-fat milk, water,
the daily soda and one cup of coffee in the morning with milk
and sugar. That sounded good to me—and healthy. Oh, yes,
there was also a big cup of tea with sugar later in the day.

If my diet was so healthy, why was I so tired. Fatigued?
Well, let's put it this way, I saw more of Oprah and Dr. Phil in
the first three months of the year than I had seen in a lifetime.
As my offices are on the first two floors of our four-story home,
I was able to go upstairs and take a nap when I needed to. And
I needed to do that daily. After making sure that I had a big

glass of water by the bed, I'd lie down and turn on the TV. Actually, I don't think I saw a complete Oprah or Dr. Phil show. It wasn't long before I was asleep. I kept complaining that I was too old to work this hard at my age. It seemed as though the last two decades had caught up with me and I was forever tired.

After dropping out of law school in 1979 and staying away from academia for one semester to first consume, and then reject, the pills, I enrolled in a masters program and then in a doctoral program and then back in law school in 1986. At that time I was forty-five years old. That was followed by the bar exam and practicing law. Then there was the major house and office fire in 1993, the move to live and work temporarily in a house that hadn't been lived in for thirteen years, practicing law on the kitchen table of the rented house. There was an extensive inventory of all of our possessions to be prepared for the insurance company. There was a house and office to be rebuilt. We returned home in 1994.

In 1998, I had turned to executive legal recruiting spending several months in a hotel in Kentucky and returning home every other weekend. Those weekends were filled with shopping, laundry and cooking. When I was back home permanently in December, I continued with the recruiting, but I still ran the law office, appeared in court on occasion, and prepared the financials on the estates. My husband had a bad medical diagnosis in 2001, and I closed the practice by the end of 2002. Those were two very busy and difficult years. All those files to close, returning almost two hundred original wills, calling in favors from local attorneys to take cases that would need attention.

Then 2003 was difficult in a different way. It was the year of the broken rib caused by a hacking cough brought home to me by my son who works as a corrections officer at the local jail. The bronchitis to go with it. And that was the year we lost a lot of close friends and relatives. One of those people was another lawyer, our golfing companion for over twenty years. He was suffering from severe complications from type 2 diabetes. Another was a long-time friend, another lawyer, who had been battling cancer for over four years. And another one was my dad who had had multiple sclerosis for sixty-two years. All three men were important support people in my life, and it seemed like one outpouring of grief after another. Now I was exhausted. Could stress and work have had such a cumulative effect that my body finally said enough is enough? I really didn't know how I was going to keep dragging my tired thirsty body through the work days.

On a positive front, I had joined a gym in 2004 and lost thirty-two pounds in about seven months. In March of 2005, my doctor was pleased. We talked about diet and exercise. She wanted me in the gym every day, in spite of the sciatic hip. I contracted to lose a total of seventy-five pounds. The nurse took blood from my arm. Good day at the doctor's office. My cholesterol numbers had been high in the past, although I never really paid attention to the warnings. After all, I had read the reports, some people with high cholesterol don't have heart attacks or strokes, and some people with low cholesterol did have strokes or heart attacks. My blood pressure had been creeping up and was of concern to the doctor, but the exercise at the gym was bringing the numbers down. As I left the doctor's office, I was hoping that the reduced weight and time in the gym had also reduced the cholesterol numbers. Hope flutters its wings in uncertain moments.

~ 2 ~

Diagnosis

A disease known is half cured.
Thomas Fuller, M.D.

It was a Saturday morning when the telephone rang. It had been eight days since the lab nurse had taken the blood sample, and I hadn't had a call from the doctor's office. Actually, I did stop to wonder whether, and hope that, my cholesterol numbers had dropped, and to worry about whether they had not, but after not hearing for a week, I assumed that things were fine. When I answered the telephone, the doctor's voice was full of concern. My doctor is very non-judgmental, patient, and calm, but today, she seemed agitated. She said that we had a problem. Of course, I jumped to the conclusion that the cholesterol was high. "The cholesterol IS very high," she said. "But what I am very concerned about is the fact that you are diabetic." Diabetic? There must have been some mistake. "Your fasting number was 389!"

Well, I didn't have a clue about diabetic numbers, but she sure seemed worried. She asked the questions. Thirst? Yes. Frequent urination? Yes. Anyone drinking the large glasses of water that I drank would be in the bathroom all the time. Fatigue? Yes. "You need to come in on Monday and we will do the Hemoglobin A1c test to see what your average blood glucose levels have been for the last three months." I asked the all-important question. "Can I do this without drugs?" "I don't think so," she said. I was a little panicked. "You don't know me very well," I said. "Just tell me what to do. I'll go back to being a vegetarian. I'll do anything. Just tell me what to do." Even as I was making these desperate pleas to avoid taking the pills, I was reminded of the scene in the movie *I Dreamed of Africa*. The mother of a boy who has been bitten by a venomous snake, says to him: "What do I do? Do I cut your arm? Do I cut your head? Tell me what to do." I also flashed on the end of the scene when her son died in her arms.

The doctor's voice cut in on my reverie: "I think you will need to open up your mind to doing things in a different way." Translation—pills for the diabetes, pills for the high cholesterol and maybe pills for the blood pressure. Then pills for the side effects or different pills to avoid the side effects. I was more afraid of the medicine than I was of the disease. The real fear of the disease would come later.

My mind wasn't going to open easily. My pill phobia had stayed with me over the years. When I had two broken toes, I refused to take medicine but sat instead with my leg hanging over the couch to relieve the pain. Even with debilitating headaches, I rarely took an aspirin. Three years ago, I had a scheduled visit to the gynecologist's office for a mammogram. I mentioned that I had a throbbing headache. "Did you ever try caffeine?" the technician asked. I hadn't had caffeine since 1979, except once in a while when I tried a can of my husband's soda to see if the caffeine would relieve a migraine. It never did.

When I got home that day, my husband's coffeepot was filled to the brim with hot coffee. In desperation, I gulped down a cup with cream and sugar. The headache went away. From then on, coffee was my "drug of choice" for treating headaches. If the coffee didn't work, I went back to the chiropractor. My rule against drugs had relaxed a little over the years. I did take an antibiotic for cellulitis when I was in law school. I did take pills for the pain of the broken rib. I did take another antibiotic for the bronchitis. My phobia now was not as generalized but more specific to pills that needed to be taken every day for the rest of my life.

Now, hearing the diagnosis of diabetes, I was scared. Refusing medicine for diabetes seemed harder than refusing medicine for high blood pressure and for high cholesterol. But I wasn't ready. I just wasn't. After all, I had been diagnosed with a "terminal" illness a quarter of a century ago, and I was still here even though I flushed the medicine down the toilet.

Again, the doctor's voice broke through my thoughts as my pill phobia was acting out, and as my mind raced to find another way to treat this new disease that had appeared out of nowhere. Had I messed up when I ate the leg of lamb and began to eat meat again? "I think this might be genetic," she said. "You have been doing things right lately." I looked at the glorious bowl of fruit on the kitchen counter. I soon understood. "I haven't. I think maybe I went mental for a while. I have been juicing lots of fruit, drinking lots of milk. Nothing but whole grains. Lots of salads. Lots of vegetables." There was a pause, then the doctor said: "Well, you should stay with just whole grains for now. We will see you on Monday to take the blood."

On the Monday, I went back to the doctor's office to have blood drawn again. My husband has a relative with the same name as mine. Her husband also had the same name as my husband. Years ago, I went to the bank to open our safe deposit and was told that it was closed. Why? I had asked. Because he died yesterday. I had to explain that that was my husband's uncle. Like the lawyers, the banks used to run through the obituaries each morning—one hoping to practice law in the form of probating an estate—the other trying to obey the law.

My husband's aunt lived close to the doctor's office and I know that they ask me for my date of birth when I sign in or call for an appointment. We have different middle initials, but

I suspect that she is a patient at my primary doctor's office, at my eye doctor's office, and at my foot doctor's office. They all ask for my date of birth. I was ready. I had had the weekend to figure out what had happened and why I had had a wrong diagnosis. The technician came at me with the needle in hand. "Hold on," I said. "Let me ask you, do you have the right Elizabeth Gemmette?" She looked at the file on the table. "Date of birth?" she asked. Same date of birth as that on the file in front of her. Middle initial? Same middle initial. It was my diabetes and I couldn't give it away. Just checking.

By the following Thursday, I had the news on the telephone. "Your Hemoglobin A1c came back at 12.9 with a Mean Blood Glucose of 342.8. You need to come in tomorrow and go over things." I asked: "Will I get out of your office without drugs?" The doctor replied, patiently: "It's your body, but I wouldn't recommend that you try to do this without medicine." I negotiated, bargained. "If I do the right things and the number comes down, will you take me off the drugs?" "I might reduce the dosage." Not the right answer. No deal. It looked as though I was going to be making this decision on my own. If I could reduce the Hemoglobin A1c with diet and exercise, how would I know that those efforts were responsible for the reduced number if I was taking pills at the same time?

Back in the doctor's office on Friday, April 1, 2005, we talked about all the important aspects of having diabetes. Check your feet every day for sores and cuts. I had noticed the sheet on the wall in front of the table reminding diabetics to take off their shoes and socks, and I was reminded of our friend who had had an amputation just before his death. Have a yearly eye exam—again, something to do with the diabetes. Follow a particular diet. That made sense, but I was surprised that the diet the doctor suggested looked like a diet tailored for anyone who wanted to eat healthy foods and lose weight.

The doctor sent me to the bathroom for a urine sample. Apparently, they were looking for protein in the urine. The doctor said that it was something else to do with the diabetes.

There was some talk about having to wait for the results, but when I complained that I hated getting the doctor's calls on a Saturday morning, the doctor said to just wait a few minutes. She came out a short time later and said that the test was just fine. I wasn't sure what bullet I had just dodged, but I was getting the idea that diabetes is very complicated and intrusive and that I was very ignorant about the disease. The doctor handed me a sheet advertising a diabetes education course at St. Clare's Hospital. "You need to get educated," she said. "You need to enroll in this program."

As she was winding down the 30-minute appointment, I looked at the doctor and asked: "Would you like me to get another doctor?" She looked at me, hesitated for a moment, then replied. "No. Actually, not many people say they are going to take charge of their own health. Most people just ask what pills they need to take."

The doctor called for a glucometer and the nurse came in and stuck my finger. He showed me the number—260! Well, we were headed in the right direction in less than one week from when I first knew that I had a problem. No more juicing for me. I was given a prescription for a blood glucose meter and test strips and lancets. I asked what numbers I was supposed to be trying to achieve. 90-120 fasting. 120-160 after meals. And how often did I need to prick my finger. Rotating: fasting, two hours after breakfast, two hours after lunch and two hours after dinner. She closed with: "Call me if the number goes over 400."

That evening, I took the prescription to the pharmacy and joined the ranks of diabetics who test their own blood glucose every day. In all truthfulness, I was close to being petrified. When I had had blood drawn at the United States Embassy in 1967 during the battery of tests they administer for immigration purposes, I had almost passed out about an hour later. I was twenty-five years old, and that was the first time I had ever had blood drawn. Well, I had matured over the years. Now when they took blood, I just looked the other way. But take the blood myself? And be ready to do that by the next day. I read the booklet over and over. All evening, I kept going over the information until I thought that I would be ready for the new blood-letting ritual about to take place. No more denial about the diagnosis. This was my disease. It didn't belong to the other Elizabeth, and I had to deal with it.

~ 3 ~

REACTIONS TO THE DIAGNOSIS

When sorrows come, they come not single spies,
But in battalions.

WILLIAM SHAKESPEARE

SOME OF MY OWN REACTIONS

What kept going through my mind when I heard the diagnosis of diabetes was, what a very bad time for this to have happened. Of course, there is never a good time for any illness to appear, but this was at a very difficult period in my life. The bad diagnosis that my husband received in 2001 was one of dementia, and, lately, things had been progressing rather quickly with his disease. Now, in 2005, I was finding it more difficult to handle all of the emotional and physical needs of my husband while at the same time meeting our financial obligations and taking on more of the physical tasks that my husband had been able to perform in the past. Fortunately, working from home made it easier for me to give him the assistance that he needed, but finding the hours I needed to put in the office was becoming impossible. Now, here was another challenge to be met and incorporated into my already busy daily activities. If I hadn't had the earlier medical scare of the "terminal heart condition," from which I made a "remarkable recovery" without continuing drug treatment, I probably would have accepted the drugs and complained about the side-effects, if, and when, they occurred. In some ways, that would have been the easier route to take, but I was conditioned to avoid drugs if at all possible. When I took time to consider the ramifications of this new disease, what came over me was an overwhelming realization that disease had seized us both. What I also realized was that one of those diseases would have to take its course, while the other might be controlled. This was the beginning of an internal dialogue about taking care of someone else and the need to take care of myself.

LACK OF SUPPORT FROM THE ONE CLOSEST TO ME

One thing that happened when I was diagnosed with diabetes was my realization that my husband could no longer support me emotionally. When I handed him a bar of Cadbury's chocolate, he would ask me if I wanted a piece. I'd say: "No, thanks, I'm diabetic." Then, when I made him a pecan pie, or a banana cream pie, or an apple pie, he'd ask if I wanted some. I'd say: "No, thanks. I'm diabetic." When we bought blueberry muffins for his breakfast, he'd ask if I wanted one. I'd say: "No, thanks. I'm diabetic." Every time I said, "I'm diabetic," he would say: "You are? I never knew that." It was very sad to realize that the person with whom I had lived for so many years, and on whom I depended to lend me support, was now unable to understand that I had diabetes. If I told him I had diabetes, he wouldn't remember that two minutes later. He would never know that I longed for him to put his arms around me and say: "I'm sorry. What can I do to help?"

OUR SON'S REACTION

Our son didn't believe that I was diabetic. It couldn't be right. There must be some mistake. He entered into the denial stage really quickly. He had been watching the changes with his father's disease, and now he was listening to his mother explain to him that she had diabetes. To him, I was the parent holding things together, and I know he was asking himself what would happen to him and to his dad if something happened to me. In some ways, this diagnosis was probably more frightening to him than it was to me because he already had information about diabetes that I didn't have. That knowledge gave him cause for concern. Working as a corrections officer for several years, he knew about diabetics and their needs for special diets, for drugs, for insulin. He knew that the nurses tested the blood glucose of diabetic prisoners and that the nurses were involved if a diabetic prisoner had symptoms suggesting that their blood glucose was too high or too low. Until he heard that I was diabetic, he absorbed the information about diabetes in a non-personal way. It was just knowledge he needed to have to perform the tasks of his job. What I noticed now was that he was coming home with stories of what the nurse had told him about diabetes, what fellow officers told him about their own diabetes, how high some of them let their numbers get—after hitting the vending machines and scoffing down candy bars. He was soliciting information to try to compare the diabetic world at large with the diabetic world of one at home, his mother.

As I began to take my blood glucose, our son would often show up to see what the numbers were. As the numbers starting dropping quickly, this seemed to give him affirmation of what he had been thinking and articulating. If I had beaten the medical drug-scare before, I would be able to do it again. He had a lot of faith in my ability to turn the diabetes around. I only hoped that I wouldn't disappoint him.

REACTIONS OF OTHER PEOPLE

It is hard to imagine that there are many people in the Untied States and other developed countries who have not heard of diabetes or who do not have some basic understanding of the serious nature of the disease. Yet, I was surprised at the ignorance many people showed toward diabetes and its complications. English friends were chatting about health issues. When the topic of my recently diagnosed diabetes came up, they were flabbergasted (gob-struck, as the English might say) when I talked about my motivation to turn the blood glucose numbers around without resorting to drugs. Just the mention of amputations and insulin injections was shocking to them. Well, they said, we have never heard of any diabetic having a limb amputated in England, and we don't know anyone who has to give themselves shots. Well, perhaps in the hand. The husband said that he once saw a woman give herself a little shot in the end of her finger, that's all. The wife said that her mother had been diabetic. Didn't make any fuss though. Took her pills. Ate what she wanted. What was even more surprising was the fact that the wife of that couple works as a receptionist in a doctor's office.

When I mentioned the diagnosis to a family member, he also commented that there was nothing to worry about. What I had was just "old-age" diabetes. Just take your medication and eat what you want. After all, it wasn't as though I had type 1 diabetes, the only type that one had to worry about.

STORIES FROM, AND ABOUT, DIABETICS

No sooner was I diagnosed with diabetes, than I started to meet and talk to people who had family members with the disease or who had the disease themselves. There were many inspirational stories about people having had the disease for many years and who had not developed any complications, about very young children taking their own blood glucose, about people managing the disease by many different methods. There were stories of hope about new studies pointing to the promise of inhaled insulin or some easy way to measure blood glucose throughout the day without the need for pricking a finger or an arm.

There were other stories from people in denial about being at risk for developing the disease. And there were stories from diabetics who refuse to test their blood glucose and who refuse to take their doctors' advice to develop healthy eating habits and incorporate exercise into their daily routines. They are in an extreme form of denial regarding the complications. They say that they feel fine. They will worry about things if, and when, they get sick. But, even in my ignorance of the complications of diabetes, I realized how dangerous it was to think like that. What I did know was that it was time for me to get down to the hard work of controlling diabetes in the most natural way that I could and to strip away any defenses of my own that might get in the way of that goal.

Part II

Diabetes Education

~ 4 ~

WHAT IS DIABETES?

Study sickness while you are well.
THOMAS FULLER, M.D.

Although I engaged in research in my professional life for many years, I did not approach this self-help "diabetes project" from a research angle. As the diabetes education program in which I participated was offered at a local hospital, I assumed that I would receive enough information to develop a plan for the control of my own diabetes. They handed out lots of materials and included talks by local physicians and a hospital pharmacist who were all knowledgeable and experienced with the diagnosis and treatment of diabetes.

Although I didn't spend time in the library pouring over medical journals, the local newspaper and several television stations bombarded me with information on a constant basis. Either those articles and news stories were rife before I had such an interest in diabetes and I hadn't been paying attention, or the topic was gaining in momentum as the numbers of diabetics swelled, probably both.

The following comments are widely-held beliefs and facts about diabetes. They were not drawn from a particular source or sources. Some of them are controversial. For instance, the genetic link to diabetes is often challenged.

How Many People Have Diabetes?

The numbers are staggering. It is believed that the number of people with diabetes exceeds 20 million. Even more shocking is the fact that over six million of those diabetics are undiagnosed. Every time you pick up a newspaper, those numbers change, always on the increase, of course.

There are many theories relating to the question of why so many diabetics are undiagnosed. Some of them are as follows:

✔ *No access to health care.* This is no longer just a concern for people from poor socio-economic backgrounds. There is a burgeoning class of elderly people who are forced to make the choice between food and drugs, or food and a visit to the doctor. As the babyboomers reach retirement age, they are finding themselves in a position of delaying their anticipated retirement dates. One reason for this delay is concern over the escalating costs of healthcare. It is believed that there are over 46 million people in the United States who are not insured for healthcare.

✔ *No symptoms to prompt a visit to the doctor.* This raises the question of whether testing is, or should be, performed on a random or routine basis and whether the testing that is performed is adequate. If the patient doesn't present with symptoms, should testing be done anyway? If so, at what age? And which test should be given? There is a cost/benefit analysis that may be skewed in the wrong direction when it comes to diagnosing diabetes.

✔ *A good test on the one morning that the fast-ing test was given.* Again, this raises the question of whether the standard fasting blood glucose test is sufficient.

✔ *A test taken when the person was in a "good stage" of diet and exercise.* These people might be called "sometime diabetics." They might account for a large number of undiagnosed diabetics. Perhaps they are yo-yo dieters who only go the doctor's office when they are in what they think of as a fairly healthy state. They have been on a diet, lost weight, and been to the gym on a regular basis. This has been going on for several months. Now they make an appointment to have blood drawn. The fasting blood glucose results are in the normal range. Next week, it's off to Bermuda, then up come the holidays, stress takes its toll, and they climb back into the overweight or obese category. Better not go back to the doctor until the weight is down.

TYPES OF DIABETES

- Gestational diabetes which shows up in pregnant women who were not previously diagnosed as diabetic.
- Type 1 diabetes, also known as juvenile diabetes because the disease is often manifested by young adulthood. Type 1 diabetics are insulin dependent and require artificial insulin.
- Type 2 diabetes. Type 2 diabetics are insulin resistant. The insulin that the pancreas makes is used in an inefficient manner. The comments to follow will address primarily type 2 diabetes.

WHAT CONTRIBUTES TO THE RISK FACTORS FOR TYPE 2 DIABETES?

- People with a family history of diabetes—this is the genetic pre-disposition theory.
- Hispanics, African-Americans, Native Americans, Asian Americans or Pacific Islanders—again, this would suggest a genetic pre-disposition for the disease.
- Women who have had a baby weighing more than nine pounds at birth.
- Anyone over the age of 45.
- Having high blood pressure.
- Having high "bad" cholesterol and low "good" cholesterol.
- Being overweight or obese.
- Poor diet.
- Inactivity.

OBESITY, POOR DIET AND INACTIVITY

Obesity, poor diet and inactivity are three crafty intertwined companions that contribute in a very interdependent way in the development of type 2 diabetes. We can't control our genetic factors, our race, or age. We can control the weight of our babies, especially with the help of the medical profession. What we can control for ourselves is what we weigh, what and how much we eat, and what kind, and how much, exercise we incorporate into our daily routines. Weight control, a healthy diet, and regular exercise work to reduce high blood glucose, high blood pressure and high "bad" cholesterol and to raise "good" cholesterol.

It is interesting to note that not all obese people are diabetic and that not all diabetics are obese. Perhaps there is some genetic factor working both to pre-dispose some thin people to diabetes and to protect others even if they are obese.

WHY DOES A PERSON WITH TYPE 2 DIABETES HAVE AN EXCESS OF BLOOD GLUCOSE?

Simply put, the body converts food into glucose which is needed for energy. A person with type 2 diabetes has a pancreas that is unable to meet the demand for insulin to transport that glucose into the cells. Again, this is known as insulin resistance. When the blood glucose is not converted for use in providing that energy, the glucose stays attached to hemoglobin and leads to hyperglycemia (diabetes).

TREATMENT OF TYPE 2 DIABETES

- Weight Loss, Diet and Exercise. Regardless of the chosen method of treatment, all patients are encouraged to take the necessary steps to lose weight, change diet, and add exercise, if those aspects of the patient's life are not already under control.
- Drugs
- Insulin/Drug Combination
- Insulin
- The Insulin Pump

TESTING FOR DIABETES

- Fasting Plasma Glucose Test. Blood is taken and tested after fasting for at least 8 hours.
- Oral Glucose Fasting Test. Blood is taken after fasting, then a sugar drink is given, and then the blood is drawn several times over the next few hours.
- The A1c Hemoglobin Test. Blood is drawn and sent to the

lab for an analysis to determine how much glucose has been stuck to the hemoglobin for the last 2-3 months. The Hemoglobin A1c number for non-diabetics is usually under 6% (average blood glucose level of 120 mg/dL or less). Diabetics are encouraged to attempt to keep good control of their blood glucose numbers to achieve a Hemoglobin A1c number under 7% (average blood glucose level of 150 mg/dL or less).

- Self-Administered Testing using a meter, lancets, and test strips. The number of times that blood is to be taken and the times that those tests are to be performed are ordered by the physician. Those tests are often taken after fasting, 1-2 hours after meals, or at bedtime. The schedule of testing depends on if, and what type of, medicine is being used by the patient.

TARGET BLOOD GLUCOSE NUMBERS

Although my doctor had told me to aim for blood glucose test results of 90-120 mg/dL fasting and 120-160 mg/dL after meals, there are different recommended ranges. As the number of diabetics goes up, the American Diabetic Association brings the recommended ranges down. The most recent range recommended by the American Diabetes Association is between 80-140 mg/dL. Test results of 70 mg/dL or below signal low blood glucose (hypoglycemia), and test results over 240 mg/dL signal high blood glucose (hyperglycemia). Both of these conditions can lead to serious health problems. Diabetics are taught how to respond to high and low blood glucose readings.

COMPLICATIONS OF DIABETES

Uncontrolled diabetes can lead to serious, severe, and life-threatening complications.

~ 5 ~

COMPLICATIONS

A good scare is worth more to a man than good advice.

EDGAR WATSON HOWE

It soon became apparent that the early symptoms of thirst, fatigue and frequent urination were mild compared with the severe complications of diabetes. On the list of reasons to reduce blood glucose numbers were heart attack, stroke, amputation, impaired vision or blindness, kidney failure and nerve damage to the bladder, the sexual organs, and the digestive system. Although I had known about diabetics enduring amputations and needing dialysis for kidney failure, I was overwhelmed by the discussion of such complications.

It seems to me that if we knew we were going to get a disease, we would pay more attention to those around us who had the disease before us. When I became a lawyer, I used to say that if I had known that I was going to law school one day, I would have paid more attention during the years when I sat in courtrooms and heard my husband argue cases. I probably sat in the back reading a novel! Now the complications of diabetes were of concern to me not just to others and I needed to pay more attention.

What could I do to avoid these complications? Simply

put, I was a time-bomb. The things to work on were controlling diabetes, reworking cholesterol numbers, regulating blood
pressure and reducing weight. In the meantime, I needed to
check my feet and eyes for damage and make sure that I
flossed after every meal.

FOOTCARE FOR DIABETICS

A local podiatrist came to one of the classes and presented a graphic slide show and told stories about the complications of diabetes that he sees in his practice. His main topics
were nerve damage causing loss of sensation and poor circula-
tion leading to foot ulcers and a slow healing process. He
noted that together these conditions could lead to cuts and
sores that are left untreated because the patient is unable to feel
the damage. This was followed by a lecture on amputation.

There was a young man in the group at the hospital
who was wheeled into the conference room in a wheelchair.
He told his story. He was having pain in his foot, so he went
to have an X-ray. The next thing he knew they were giving him
an insulin shot. His foot was badly crushed but because he had
advanced untreated diabetes, he was unable to feel what others would have experienced as excruciating pain. That level of
pain would have alerted him much sooner to the damage to his
foot.

One piece of advice from the nurse was to wear slippers in the house at all times. That didn't really seem that necessary. We have a very clean house, no children leaving toys
on the floor, and no reason to believe that I would cut my feet.
Anyway, I shopped for slippers and began to wear them
around the house as soon as I got out of bed in the morning,
even to go to the bathroom in the night.

About a week later, I entered the kitchen in the morning and noticed a silver bowl on the counter-top. I looked
inside and saw purple hazy pieces that looked like candy. As

I looked closer, I realized that this was a dish full of broken glass. My husband had dropped a large purple Pyrex dish on the kitchen floor during the night. Although he had picked up the larger pieces, it goes without saying that there were still small pieces of glass scattered around the floor. Slippers for everyone—diabetic or not!

The nurse recommended a foot doctor. Why? Well, to see if you have any loss of feeling or any nerve damage—to make sure that I didn't end up like the young man in the wheelchair. My doctor's office responded that I didn't need a foot doctor, yet! It turned out that my co-pay for a foot doctor under my HMO was $40.00. The charge to have my toenails cut was $40.00. I was in.

In the waiting room at the podiatrist's office, I sat next to a woman and started up a conversation. We were talking about why we were there when she said that she had had all kinds of infections on her feet. "From what?" I asked. "Well," she said, "I was cutting my toenails with the garden shears." As I sat in the doctor's chair waiting to get my toenails cut, I kept glancing at the rug. I had taken my shoes and socks off and walked across the rug to the chair. Now I had to get back across that rug to my shoes. What creatures were crawling on that carpet? I decided then that when I got my toenails cut, I would leave my socks on and wear them to and from the chair. As well as cutting my toenails, the doctor did the tests for damage from the diabetes. There was no damage to my feet. The recommendation from all of the professionals was to check the bottom of my feet every day for cuts or sores.

There was talk about buying and wearing socks made especially for diabetics. Unable to find a suitable sock locally, I ordered them from the FootSmart® catalogue. When they arrived, I tried a pair on. They were so embracing—warm, seam free, with terry linings. I would wear them forever, even if I controlled the diabetes!

EYE CARE FOR DIABETICS

Both my doctor and the nurse had insisted on an annual eye exam. The nurse spent time stressing the fact that diabetics are at risk for going blind. I had planned to make an appointment fairly soon after the diagnosis, but I was prompted to pick up the phone rather quickly and schedule the check up immediately. Quite suddenly, I developed a bad case of blurred vision. Oddly enough, I had had no problems with my eyesight before the diagnosis of diabetes, but within a couple of weeks my vision was so blurred that I was having a problem seeing faces. I borrowed my husband's glasses when I drove the car. It was rather frightening. I wondered if it was in my head, not really in my eyes.

The eye doctor gave me more good news. No damage. I asked him if he thought the blurred vision would go away. The dietician had said that sometimes the doctor doesn't change the prescription for a few months to see what happens if the blood glucose numbers go down. No, he said, he thought my eyesight would not get any better.

I bought progressive lenses and was pleased to be able to drive the car, work on the computer and read a book with one pair of glasses. I never wore the reading glasses that I bought at the same time. It did make me very nervous to think that the changes to my vision were a sign of bad things to come, even though there was no damage to my eyes according to the doctor. Then a strange thing happened, my eyesight started changing again. After a few weeks had passed, my eyesight was back to where it had been before the diagnosis. I could see faces clearly again, and I could see to drive without glasses. The progressive lenses still worked, but I was wearing them in the wrong position to accommodate the changes in my eyesight. I made another appointment with the eye doctor. Sure enough, he re-examined my eyes and had to change the prescription to reflect the positive changes in my vision.

DENTAL CARE FOR DIABETICS

My routine dental appointment was already scheduled, and flossing had been on the agenda for many years, but now I made sure I never missed—an appointment or flossing. The dental appointment showed no gum disease.

So for now, the feet, eyes and teeth were checked and showed no damage from the diabetes. I learned later that the urine test that they had taken at my doctor's office to check for protein or microalbumin was performed to determine whether there was any damage to the blood vessels in the kidneys. Damage to the blood vessels in the kidneys can lead to diabetic nephropathy and this, in turn, can cause kidney failure. Now that I knew more about the complications of diabetes, I had had "a good scare," and I knew that I had to work on controlling the blood glucose as quickly and effectively as possible.

~ 6 ~

DIET AND EXERCISE

To learn new habits is everything, for it is to reach the substance of life. Life is but a tissue of habits.

HENRI FRÉDÉRIC AMIEL

One hour with a nutritionist who ran the diabetes program at the local hospital was the most valuable hour I could have spent on diabetes education. Who knew it was so simple! All those years of messing with this diet and that diet. There were lots of diets: Counting points in the Weight Watchers® program (I could always eke out enough points for a candy bar or a hamburger at a fast-food restaurant). Giving up carbs on the Atkins Diet (never felt sure about that one, especially with the mixed medical reviews). Meals centered around just carbs or just protein on Suzanne Somers diet (I developed a bad case of the shakes by the second day and stuffed anything I could find into my mouth in panic). No starches at first and then the introduction of limited starches at LA Weight Loss® Center (sick of protein and craving carbs within the first week). Let's not forget the boiled egg diet, the cabbage soup diet, the rice diet and many other diets, the names of which I have now forgotten.

There are many people who swear by all of the diets

mentioned above, and everyone needs to seek out solutions to their own dietary needs and tolerance for different ways of eating. What struck me now was that the plan that I was to follow was very similar to the one that used to be in place at Weight Watchers® many years ago. The one that never worked for me then, but would work for me now. It had to!

Using the *Exchange Lists for Meal Planning* (2003) prepared by the American Diabetes Association and the American Dietetic Association, the nutritionist made a list of what units I should consume:

> 11 carbohydrate units—15 grams of carbohydrates each (starches, fruits, milk, and treats)
> 6 meat units
> 3 vegetable units
> 3-4 fat units

They were to be consumed in the following manner:

Breakfast:	3 Carbs, 1 Meat, 1 Fat
Lunch:	3 Carbs, 1 1/2 Nonstarchy Vegetables, 2 Meat, 1 Fat
Dinner:	4 Carbs, 1 1/2 Nonstarchy Vegetables, 3 Meat, 1-2 Fat
Extra:	1 Carb

This combination of foods would make up approximately 1400 calories.

The first thing I did was to make up a template and take it to Office Max. For a few dollars, they produced several hundred 4" x 2" cards with the following information printed on them:

DATE: WEIGHT:

Starch (7)
Fruit (2)
Milk (2)

Protein (6)
Fat (3-4)
Vegetables (3)

Vitamin: Water:

BP: _____
BG: _____ F AB AL AD
        (Fasting, After Breakfast, After Lunch,
                    After Dinner)

Those cards became invaluable in my learning process and in re-vamping my diet to eat less, eat well, and eat at prescribed times. It soon became second nature to me to know what to eat at each meal, but those cards really helped me to get the plan in place initially. Each day, I left one dated card on my desk, then took it with me to the gym to record the blood pressure and carried it in my pocketbook when we went out to eat. Putting a check mark against each exchange as it was eaten kept me honest and reminded me of what I had consumed as each day wore on. Writing down blood pressure numbers at the gym and recording the blood glucose after taking it on a rotating basis provided a good review of progress to that point. In addition to the cards, I kept a yellow pad and recorded the blood glucose numbers daily.

After a few weeks, I began to record both my blood glucose and blood pressure numbers in a short-hand notebook. I wrote fourteen dates down the left-hand side of each page. Each page was marked at the top with Blood Glucose on the left and Blood Pressure on the right. At the end of the fourteen days, I recorded the fourteen day average and the thirty day average for the blood glucose.

In spite of my sciatic hip, my doctor had said: "Every day. I want you in the gym every day." The nurse who was part of the staff in the diabetes program also insisted on exercise every day and encouraged increasing time on the bike and the repetitions on the machines and adding walks before and/or after meals. At first, I rode a stationary bike for about fifteen minutes and did one set of ten repetitions on five leg machines, and one set of ten repetitions with weights for the arms. Over the next few weeks, I increased the time on the bike to thirty minutes and increased the repetitions for the leg and arm exercises to two sets of ten and added a ball exercise to work the stomach and the butt—again, two sets of ten. One advantage of my gym, which is attached to a rehabilitation center, is that staff members are more than willing to accommodate a request for a blood pressure reading.

The exercise time had increased, the diet was becoming second-nature, the blood glucose numbers were coming down, the blood pressure was in a very good range, and the weight was dropping quickly. What I was curious about was whether the cholesterol was also changing in the right direction. That would have to wait. One thing that I could do right now was to follow up on a suggestion made by the dietician. She had made the comment that if I was going to try to control diabetes with diet and exercise alone without the use of medicine, then I might want to look at the Glycemic Index. Choices of foods with a low Glycemic Index were said to help with maintaining low blood glucose. My immediate goal was to look at the Glycemic Index and to try to incorporate useful information into my food choices.

Part III

More About Diet

~ 7 ~

Fruit, Milk, Protein, and Starches

But the truth was, we'd started this—we'd started counting individual berries, keeping a record by bush, and we couldn't stop. . . . We saved our 200,000th blueberry and set it on the front windowsill at Barra, where it slowly dried.
LAURA WATERMAN

Reflections on My Diet

It was while I was riding the bike at the gym that I read *Losing the Garden* by Laura Waterman. The idea of someone counting every blueberry they harvested seemed to me the ultimate illustration of an obsessive compulsive disorder. That caused me to question my own interest in diet, in counting servings, in taking blood samples at the right moment, in refining the diet suggested by the nutritionist and in avoiding many foods. Many of the foods that I avoided were allowed by the American Diabetes Association and The American Dietetic Association in their publication *Exchange Lists for Meal Planning* (2003).

As I alluded to in the Introduction to this book, I purchased only three books as reference tools to aid me in my quest for health. Those books are *The G-Index Diet* by Richard N. Podell, M.D., F.A.C.P. (1993), *Reversing Diabetes* by Julian Whitaker, M.D. (2001), and *The New Glucose Revolution* by Brand-Miller, et al. (2003). These books will be referred to in the next few chapters.

On reflecting on what I am compulsive about in terms of the diet, I would say that I am most compulsive about fruit, milk, protein and starches—sometimes in exchange choices, always in portion sizes.

PORTION CONTROL AND FOOD CHOICES

The *Exchange Lists for Meal Planning* (2003) is a valuable reference tool for serving sizes. After all, one of the lessons to be learned in any diet is portion control, and I had known for a long time that I had to learn this lesson if I was going to lose weight and keep it off. In studying the exchange lists, I was surprised to see the inclusion of such items as sugar-frosted cereal, raisin bread, hot dog buns, french-fried potatoes, baked and mashed potatoes, doughnuts, cake, ice cream and pumpkin pie. Most of the foods that I instinctively eschewed showed up on the Starch List and in the Sweets, Desserts, and Other Carbohydrates List of the *Exchange Lists for Meal Planning* (2003, 8-11, 16-19).

This was where I had to make a very serious and important decision. Did I want to take the path that lead to choosing a cookie instead of one serving of oatmeal and the fat serving to make that oatmeal tasty? Or to choose a 2 ounce piece of cake instead of the bread for a sandwich and the fat to put on that bread. Or to choose 1/6 of an 8-inch two-crust pie and use up three of my carbohydrate servings and 2/3 of the day's fat? In the diabetes workshop at the hospital, it was pointed out that if you wanted potato chips, you could have potato chips. Just ten instead of a slice of bread. What kind of nutritional trade-off was that?

It is part of our culture to want what we want when we want it. Couple that with the old adage: "A little won't hurt you," and we are on the proverbial slippery slope. Maybe a little of those sugary snacks would hurt me now that I was diabetic. What I really needed was the will-power to resist cravings for unhealthy food. Giving in to cravings might lead me into temptation and send me on that slippery slope to diet failure and make my goal of controlling my diabetes solely with diet and exercise unreachable. If I was developing compulsions to avoid unhealthy foods altogether, that was good. Sometimes compulsions are healthy tools.

FRUIT

Daily Servings—2
Portions—4 oz. of fresh fruit or 1/2 cup fresh juice
Choices—Guided by the Glycemic Index

I turned to the *Exchange Lists for Meal Planning* for portion sizes for fruits (2003, 12-13) and to *The G-Index Diet* for information on which fruits are least likely to raise blood glucose levels sharply (Podell 1993, 293-294). Podell rates foods on a scale of 1-4, with 1 and 2 being the most desirable low glycemic foods and 4 being the least desirable (1993, 14). Based on the information provided by Podell, I do not eat bananas, kiwis, mangos, pineapples, or raisins. There are so many fruits that have low numbers on the Glycemic Index that it is not difficult to eliminate these other fruits that have a tendency to raise blood glucose levels rapidly. Every day, I have 4 ounces of orange juice or grapefruit juice or a combination of orange juice and grapefruit juice and choose one other fruit from the low-glycemic list.

MILK

Daily Servings—2
Portions—1 cup of 1% milk or 1 cup of buttermilk or 2/3 cup
of plain low-fat yogurt
Choices—Two of any combination of low-fat milk, buttermilk,
or yogurt

Milk is the easiest food category to deal with. Most
days, I have two cups of 1% milk. Occasionally, I consume 2/3
of a cup of low-fat yogurt as part of those milk exchanges.
Buttermilk is also an option. Although the nutritionist lumped
milk, fruit and starches under carbohydrates and mentioned
that if I chose not to drink the milk or eat the fruit, I could have
more bread, or pasta, or other grains, I do not omit the allowed
servings of fruit or milk on any day.

PROTEIN

Daily Servings—6
Portions—Basically, serving sizes are 1 oz. of cheese,
fish, meat, or poultry; or
3 slices of bacon; or
1 tablespoon of peanut butter; or
1 egg; or
2 oz. of ricotta cheese; or
1/4 cup of low-fat cottage cheese; or
2 tablespooons of grated Parmesan cheese; or
1 oz. of turkey sausage; or
2 sardines; or
4 oz. of tofu.
Beans, peas and lentils are a little tricky. They are an excellent source of protein, but 1/2 cup cooked counts as both a
protein and a starch

Choices—Any combination of the above foods.

Protein is also easy to incorporate into the diet. The *Exchange Lists for Meal Planning* includes protein of all kinds under the Meat and Meat Substitutes List grouping items under very lean, lean, medium fat, and high fat exchanges (2003, 22-27).

I am compulsive about serving sizes and the number of servings that I consume in the protein category, but I do not obsess about whether I am consuming items from the very lean, lean, medium fat or high fat categories. As I only consume six protein servings a day, it is unlikely that I am making poor choices. Most of the cheese that I consume is 50% fat-free. An ounce of this is usually included with my breakfast oatmeal. I do like peanut butter and use one tablespoon almost every day. How much damage can I do with four ounces of meat on a day in which I choose all high fat exchanges compared with a diet of eggs and bacon for breakfast, a hamburger for lunch and an eight-ounce steak for dinner. Besides, I include fish and poultry in my choices on a frequent basis which makes my exposure to meat even more limited.

STARCHES

Daily Servings—5 (modified from the 7 allowed)
Portions—Each portion consists of 15 grams of carbohydrate
Choices—Guided by the Glycemic Index

Starches present the most difficult challenge to a diabetic, and there are many starches that I now avoid completely. Those starches include white potatoes, cold cereal, most rice and white bread. At the moment, my servings are very controlled and tend to be rather limited, most often selected from the following list: coucous, oatmeal, whole wheat and white pasta, stoneground whole-wheat, pumpernickel, and rye bread, taco shells, and Wasa® crackers (Podell 1993, 280-285; *Exchange Lists for Meal Planning* [2003, 8-9]). Wasa Crackers are not in the *Exchange Lists for Meal Planning* but do conform to the recommenced carbohydrate serving of fifteen grams per serving, in this case 1 1/2 crackers.

There are other starches that I am cautious about eating but might try adding to the diet later. Those starches are sweet potatoes or yams, whole wheat English muffins, buckwheat pancakes, and Basmati rice.

My diet now consists of two fruit servings, two milk servings and six protein servings. It also includes five starch servings, modified from the seven allowed. Although I am compulsive about my choices in the fruit and starch servings, and precise about portion control in the fruit, milk, protein and starch servings, I am not compulsive about serving sizes for non-starchy vegetables and fat. This is explained in the next chapter.

~ 8 ~

Vegetables, Fats, and Alcohol

Yum, Yum, Pig's Bum.
If I have a party, you won't come.
Bread without butter,
Tea without sugar.
Yum, Yum, Pig's Bum.

Anonymous

Vegetables

The suspect non-starchy vegetables that might have a tendency to raise blood glucose levels are beets, carrots, carrot juice, snow peas, and turnips. Again, there are enough other vegetables to choose from, and I never did like beets or turnips. I must confess that my compulsion to eat right is undermined by my newly-found love of frozen pea pods. Peapods are counted as a vegetable, but green peas are counted as both a starch and a vegetable. By using peapods, there is a net saving of one starch, and I do like peas enough to go to a food with a slightly higher Glycemic Index here (Podell, 1993, 290-292).

Servings are basically 1/2 cup cooked or 1 cup raw or 5 grams of carbohydrate (*Exchange Lists for Meal Planning*, 2003, 20-21). As my diet calls for 3 vegetable exchanges, and as vegetables are consumed mostly at lunch and at dinner, my servings tend to be about 3/4 cup cooked or 1 1/2 cups raw for each meal. My measurements here are not precise, but if I am pouring out frozen vegetables, I do note the carbohydrates for their serving size and adjust the measurement to equal about 7-8 carbohydrates per meal. If I include vegetables in a recipe, I tend to give a quick glance at the ingredients and adjust additional vegetables at lunch or dinner, if necessary. One popular meal of mine includes celery for lunch. As the celery included in that meal tends to be less than 1 1/2 servings of vegetables, I do not fret about having a little over on the vegetable portion with the dinnertime meal.

As noted earlier, legumes (beans, peas and lentils) are counted as both a starch and a protein. Serving sizes are 1/2 cup of cooked beans, peas and lentils, except for lima beans which have a serving size of 2/3 cup (*Exchange Lists for Meal Planning*, 2003, 11). They all carry a low Glycemic Index (Podell, 1993, 282).

Starchy vegetables include baked beans, corn, corn on the cob, green peas, potatoes, squash and yams or sweet potatoes (*Exchange Lists for Meal Planning*, 1993, 10). As these starchy vegetables, except for peas and yams, all carry a high Glycemic Index, I do not include them in my diet. As mentioned before, peas carry a low Glycemic Index, but they do count as both a starch and a vegetable. Yams and sweet potatoes are low on the Glycemic Index and are on my "to try later" list. So are the boiled potatoes, but although Podell recommends boiling rather than baking pototoes, even boiled pototes are only "moderately desirable" on the Glycemic Index, and I am not sure whether I want to try them or not (Podell, 1993, 62-63, 282). If I consume green peas, I make a starch adjustment.

FATS

It is probably surprising to hear me say that I do not measure the fat that goes into my diet. Let me explain. The only added fats that I use are as follows:

Avocado
Benecol® Light
Olive Oil
Low-Fat Mayonnaise
Low-Fat Sour Cream

Before my doctor and I knew that I was diabetic, she had recommended Benecol® to reduce cholesterol. When I asked the dietician at the hospital how Benecol® fits into the food program for diabetics, she wasn't really sure. When I asked my doctor she said to use it as directed. The instructions on the Bencol® are to use AT LEAST two tablespoons per day. No, I do not mean that that gives me license to slather the spread on bread and vegetables. What I do mean is that two tablespoons go a long way. Benecol® is the added fat that I use for most meals. I do not feel the urge to measure, especially as I now use Benecol® Light with only fifty calories for a full tablespoon. If I use two tablespoons of Benecol® and add a teaspoon of olive oil or a tablespoon of low-fat mayonnaise, each with 40-50 calories per serving, I am really using the calorie equivalent of three fats. As I am allowed 3-4 per day, I am within the range. Low-fat sour cream and avocado are rare treats.

ALCOHOL

Alcohol is a very controversial topic and has special importance when the discussion turns to the inclusion of alcohol in the diets of diabetics. The dietician asked if I drank alcohol. I said that I do two or three times a week if we are eating in a restaurant. For the most part, I do not drink at home. She thought about this for a moment, and then she responded that diabetics have to be careful with alcohol because alcohol reduces blood glucose. Brand-Miller et al. confirm that alcohol lowers blood glucose levels and they carry a warning that this can sometimes be dangerous for diabetics. They also recommend only moderate intake of alcohol (2003, 250). The dietician had gone on to say that for those patients on drug treatment there was a risk that the drugs and the alcohol together would reduce the blood glucose to unsafe levels—there was a chance of a hypoglycemic attack. Then she reflected that as I was going to try to reduce the blood glucose numbers without drugs, I wouldn't run into this problem with both drugs and alcohol combining to reduce blood glucose to dangerous levels. However, she did recommend that alcohol be consumed with a meal. When I discussed with my doctor the idea of adding a drink with dinner each evening, she said that this might not be a bad idea as it might help with reducing "bad" cholesterol.

Whitaker deals with the question of whether or not diabetics should drink alcohol. "For more than twenty years we've known that people who drink moderate amounts of wine, beer, and spirits have increased levels of protective HDL cholesterol and a reduced risk of heart attack." And "[w]e now know that rather than worsening the diabetic condition, judicious use of alcohol actually improves insulin sensitivity." He gives the necessary warning: "Alcohol is a double-edged sword. The majority of people who drink do so in moderation and clearly derive benefits from it." He goes on to note: "Be aware, however, that habitual abuse of alcohol affects roughly 10% of the drinking population and requires treatment" (2001, 126-127).

As I had decided to add one drink a day, the dilemma was what to drink. It is noted in the *Exchange Lists for Meal*

Planning that the choices for women are one 12 ounce beer, one 5-ounce glass of wine or 1 1/2 ounces of hard liquor, while men are allowed two drinks per day (2003, 4). Both red wine and white wine have given me severe headaches in the past, and I wasn't willing to take a chance on that. I tried beer a couple of times with my meal but found that my blood glucose tended to be elevated afterwards. Finally, I settled on one serving, 3 tablespoons, of gin served with 4 ounces of fresh-squeezed orange juice, or fresh-squeezed grapefruit juice, or a combination of both fresh-squeezed orange and fresh-squeezed grapefruit juice.

The question was how to count alcohol in the diet. *The Exchange Lists for Meal Planning* carried a recommendation not to omit food from the meal plan when alcohol is consumed as alcohol is considered an addition, rather than a replacement (2003, 4). The dietician also said that I should make this an addition, not a substitution. But, I was a little concerned about calories. What I decided to do was to use two of the carbohydrate exchanges for the alcohol, in effect using about the same number of calories for the alcohol as I was giving up in carbohydrates. This left my meal plan just one carbohydrate short of the recommendations in the *Exchange Lists for Meal Planning* (2003, 1). This seemed to be a fair trade, especially as all of my exchanges were of the healthy variety. It would not benefit too much if I added back the one carbohydrate as a sugar-laden food such as a small portion of cookies, ice cream or cake. What mattered to me now was not the missed exchange but keeping wasted calories and unhealthy calories out of my diet. In this vein, there was no place in my diet for butter and there was no place for sugar.

~ 9 ~

DIET PRODUCTS, SUGAR SUBSTITUTES, AND SUGAR

Things sweet to taste prove in digestion sour.
WILLIAM SHAKESPEARE

The following diet products, sugar substitutes, and sugar-substitute enhanced foods are allowed as free foods or limited foods in the *Exchange Lists for Meal Planning* (2003, 32-33). Limited foods are those items that have a serving size listed beside them and are limited to 3 servings a day spread throughout the day:

Sugar-Free Foods

Candy, hard, sugar free	1 candy
Gelatin dessert, sugar-free	
Gum, sugar-free	
Sugar substitutes	
Syrup, sugar free	2 Tbsp.

Sugar-Free Drinks

Diet soft drinks, sugar free
Drink mixes, sugar free
Tonic water, sugar-free

*The sugar-free items on this list contain

sugar substitutes. Sugar substitutes show
up as a separate listing. The sugar substitutes   that   the   American   Diabetes
Association cites the FDA as approving as
safe for use are as follows:

Equal ® (aspartame)
Splenda ® (sucralose)
Sprinkle Sweet ® (saccharin)
Sweet One ® (acesulfame K)
Sweet-10 ® (saccharin)
Sugar Twin ® (saccharin)
Sweet 'N Low ® (saccharin)

My own experience with sugar substitutes is the same
as that experienced in response to drinking wines, both red
and white. Sugar substitutes produce severe headaches. There
was a time when I took tea to bed in the evening and used a
sugar substitute as a sweetener. It took a long time before I
realized that the band headache that I had each morning was
caused by the sugar substitute that I had added to my tea the
night before. To me, the taste of sweetened tea was not worth
the discomfort and the pain.

Although the FDA has said that the sugar substitutes
listed above are safe for use, there are those who would dis-
agree. Whitaker has a lengthy discussion of sugar substitutes
and their link to many side effects, including, but not limited to
headache, vision loss, seizures, mood disorders, other nervous
problems and tumors. More importantly, he points out that
sucralose (Splenda) was shown in one small study to raise levels of HbAlc. His comment is of real concern for diabetics:
"This suggests that it may worsen the diabetic condition. Until
all safety questions are cleared up, stay away from sucralose"
(2001, 124-126). As you might have guessed, I do not use sugar
substitutes. I do not use sugar, except that which occurs natu-
rally in fruit and milk products in the form of fructose and lac-
tose.

In one class at the hospital, the instructor asked the question: "What was once forbidden in the diets of diabetics, but is now allowed?" The answer was SUGAR. Sugar shows up on the *Exchange Lists for Meal Planning* as one tablespoon equaling one carbohydrate (2003, 19). Without belaboring the point too much, let that one carbohydrate that I am missing from my diet be a missed serving of one tablespoon of sugar! That tablespoon of sugar would add nothing nutritionally and might have a very bad outcome if consumed.

During one of our classes at the hospital, one of the former participants came in to speak. He told the group that if anyone had an urge for chocolate, they should just eat the real thing. After all, who knew what those sugar-substitutes might do to you. Do we really want to take a chance with a box of real chocolates, either? Chocolates are like the old potato chip advertisement: Bet you can't eat just one.

Yes, I am human. It occurred to me at the beginning of this experiment that I could give up a slice of bread and add sugar to my coffee. The problem with this idea is the same as mentioned earlier. Should I add a doughnut for breakfast and use up two more carbohydrates and two fats. And how about a piece of frosted cake in the afternoon for two more carbohydrates and one more fat. Sugar in my coffee, a doughnut and a piece of frosted cake. There go 5 carbohydrates and 3 fats—my limit for the day.

Podell discusses the consumption of sugar and sugar substitutes, noting: "Many people find sugar addictive. The more they eat, the more they want—and the more they must consume before they can find that sweet taste again" (1993, 64). That certainly captures my own addiction to fructose in those large glasses of fruit juice and the end result of adding soda in the afternoons. I was addicted to sugar for a very short time. I became diabetic. I will not experiment with dangerous sugar and sugar substitutes.

When I mentioned that I had slipped into drinking one soda in the afternoon to help with my raging thirst, my doctor asked if it was diet soda. No, it wasn't. She suggested that I try diet soda. Podell makes a similar comment about artificial sweeteners as he does about sugar: "[C]onsuming large amounts of sweetened food or drink perpetuates the desire for sweets. Abstaining from sweets, both artificial and natural, reduces that desire after several weeks—a major blessing for dieters" (1993, 64). Not only did I not want the addiction, I did not want the headaches.

Podell's comments confirm my own concern about sugar and the built-in opportunity to have one's cake and eat it too. Let's just say that I have very good will-power in follow-ing a rigid diet program. If the notion of adding just a bit of the "tasty stuff" gets back into my diet, my mouth, and my head, where would I end up? To me, it's like saying to an alcoholic: "One drink won't hurt you." We all know the answer to that. It also seems to me that it is insulting to us if every diet that comes along has some provision to let us eat what we like the most—even if that food is the food to which we are addicted.

So reintroducing diet products, sugar substitutes and sugar is not on my list of things to do. The very idea of doing that leaves a sour taste in my mouth. If I tried to use them as a reward for lowering blood glucose numbers, they might act as a punishment. What I am looking forward to is the reward of moving toward a healthy state. If I am over-compulsive, if I am too hard on myself, if I am giving up some treats which really wouldn't hurt me, what does that matter. My goal is not to cheat the system, my goal is not to squeeze out every taste sensation that I desire. My only goal is to find my way back to health.

Part IV

Reaping the Rewards

~ 10 ~

Positive Progress

*Trouble will come soon enough, and when he
does, come receive him as pleasantly as possible.
Like the tax-collector, he is a disagreeable chap to
have in one's house, but the more amiably you
greet him the sooner he will go away.*

ARTEMUS WARD

As the days turned to weeks, and the weeks to months, I became more comfortable with testing my own blood glucose. At first, I hated the idea of sticking my finger. After I returned home from the drug store with the kit, I called my doctor's office and asked if I was supposed to test once a week. No, once a day. Rotating: fasting, two hours after breakfast, two hours after lunch and two hours after dinner. I knew it was rotating, but I was hoping that it was once a week, not once a day. The doctor must have reflected that there was yet another reluctant participant in self-care. That reluctance was only fleeting.

One thing that is really useful for diabetics is the ability to self-monitor the disease. It is now part of my daily routine and something that I enjoy. That's right, enjoy. It gives me fast feedback on how certain foods and exercise and stress affect my readings. This allows me to change and modify habits accordingly. I attend the gym regularly and try to work-out on a daily basis. On the occasional days that the gym is closed, I add a long walk that day or work in the garden. With my doctor's approval, I have modified the diet slightly, but I have not cheated once by eating foods that are not permitted or by eating portions that are not controlled.

The dietician's suggestion that I should look at the Glycemic Index if I wanted to try to do this without medicine was invaluable. As I indicated earlier, I restricted my choice of foods further than required by the *American Diabetes Exchange Lists*. If I do get tempted to let foods into the diet that are allowed but that I have omitted, I only have to look at my results so far.

Let me review the blood glucose numbers from April 2nd through July 8th reading left to right:

4/2/05	291	4/3/05	280	4/4/05	279
4/5/05	211	4/6/05	295	4/7/05	290
4/8/05	285	4/9/05	320	4/10/05	158
4/11/05	214	4/12/00	273	4/13/05	270
4/14/05	217	4/15/05	253	4/16/05	179
4/17/05	163	4/18/05	189	4/19/05	205
4/20/05	148	4/21/05	155	4/22/05	165
4/23/05	147	4/24/05	150	4/25/05	126
4/26/05	167	4/27/05	131	4/28/05	132
4/29/05	124	4/30/05	142	5/1/05	120
5/2/05	144	5/3/05	131	5/4/05	132
5/5/05	125	5/6/05	139	5/7/05	142
5/8/05	117	5/9/05	97	5/10/05	130
5/11/05	140	5/12/00	122	5/13/05	120
5/14/05	154	5/15/05	146	5/16/05	115
5/17/05	101	5/18/05	132	5/19/05	128
5/20/05	108	5/21/05	102	5/22/05	133
5/23/05	107	5/24/05	113	5/25/05	104
5/26/05	111	5/27/05	142	5/28/05	117
5/29/05	100	5/30/05	104	5/31/05	114
6/1/05	115	6/2/05	108	6/3/05	132
6/4/05	118	6/5/05	116	6/6/05	113

6/7/05	122	6/8/05	117	6/9/05	132
6/10/05	113	6/11/05	100	6/12/05	107
6/13/05	100	6/14/05	142	6/15/05	129
6/16/05	101	6/17/05	86	6/18/05	121
6/19/05	109	6/20/05	104	6/21/05	114
6/22/05	109	6/23/05	112	6/24/05	108
6/25/05	106	6/26/05	126	6/27/05	112
6/28/05	105	6/29/05	89	6/30/05	108
7/1/05	96	7/2/05	108	7/3/05	115
7/4/05	106	7/5/05	106	7/6/06	104
7/7/05	81	7/8/05	127		

Here are the 14-day and 30-day averages:

	14 Day Average	30 Day Average
4/2/05 - 4/15/05	268	268
4/16/05 - 4/29/05	156	211
4/30/05 - 5/13/05	129	151
5/14/05 - 5/27/05	121	125
5/28/05 - 6/10/05	116	119
6/11/05 - 6/24/05	110	114
6/25/05 - 7/8/05	106	109

Here are the high and low numbers for the 14-day periods:

	High	Low
4/2/05 - 4/15/05	320	158
4/16/05 - 4/29/05	205	124
4/30/05 - 5/13/05	144	97
5/14/05 - 5/27/05	154	102
5/28/05 - 6/10/05	132	100
6/11/05 - 6/24/05	142	86
6/25/05 - 7/8/05	126	81

Some observations on the numbers for the first three months. Once I stopped juicing and drinking lots of milk and eating lots of salads and vegetables, the number dropped from the fasting number of 389 in March to the fasting number obtained by the nurse on April 1st of 260. That change occurred in less than a week after changing my dietary habits. My 14-day averages from that date on continued to drop. As you can see, the average numbers dropped significantly: 268, to 156, to 129, to 121, to 116, to 110, to 106 in just over three months.

Looking at the individual numbers for the first three months, we see that they also dropped rapidly, both on the high end and on the low end. The results were very rewarding. The question for me was what had caused such a rapid decline in blood glucose.

Of the three elements working to reduce the blood glucose numbers—diet, exercise, and weight loss—I have to believe that the immediate benefit came from changing the diet. The rapid drop in blood glucose levels was remarkable. This is especially true when you consider that what I call the "old bad blood" takes two to three months to be replaced. For me the question became whether my blood from April 1st would have produced numbers around 110 immediately just by the change in diet if it were not for the fact that the old blood was still hanging around and only slowly being leeched out. Now we were past the 3-month mark, and I hoped that the numbers I was now recording would be about the same as the months progressed.

In referring to my old notes for blood glucose numbers, I noticed that I had also kept blood pressure readings on a fairly consistent basis from April 16, 2005 through May 23, 2005. They are as follows reading left to right:

4/16/05	138/80	4/17/05	135/80
4/18/05	-0-	4/19/05	128/72
4/20/05	-0-	4/21/05	144/76
4/22/05	-0-	4/23/05	137/76
4/24/05	132/80	4/25/05	136/86
4/26/05	124/74	4/27/05	138/78
4/28/05	120/78	4/29/05	138/80
4/30/05	124/75	5/1/05	123/75

5/2/05	134/76	5/3/05	124/78
5/4/05	-0-	5/5/05	128/84
5/6/05	118/70	5/7/05	122/76
5/08/05	120/78	5/9/05	130/76
5/10/05	128/68	5/11/05	130/78
5/12/00	132/74	5/13/05	112/70
5/14/05	123/80	5/15/05	-0-
5/16/05	122/68	5/17/05	126/68
5/18/05	-0-	5/19/05	114/62
5/20/05	-0-	5/21/05	130/75
5/22/05	118/62	5/23/05	128/68

After May 23rd, the blood pressure recordings become sparser. I suppose that I had dropped one compulsion anyway—the need to monitor blood pressure on a daily basis. The numbers were coming in consistently below the 130/80 recommended by the various professionals with whom I had come into contact in the recent months. The numbers that were recorded on certain days from May 24th through July 8th were as follows: 110/78, 120/68, 124/72, 108/68, 118/65, 128/70, 112/68, 130/70, 126/78, 130/80, 112/70, 112/78, 120/70 and 129/70.

Things were looking good with the blood glucose and the blood pressure numbers. New cholesterol readings and the all-important Hemoglobin A1c to measure my blood glucose average for a period of two to three months would have to wait a little longer.

~ 11 ~

A Full Vasovagal, Without Cream Cheese

How often have I said to you that when you have eliminated the impossible, whatever remains, however improbable, must be the truth?
Sir Arthur Conan Doyle

It was September 9th, a Saturday, just over five months since the doctor had given me the diagnosis of diabetes. It was about a month or so away from my scheduled appointment for a follow-up Hemoglobin A1c. It was also two weeks away from the scheduled visit of friends from England. They were staying from Friday through Tuesday morning, then going to Boston for a few days, then coming back again to stay from Friday through Tuesday morning.

During the summer, I like to be outside in the garden or taking long walks. So, I start heavy cleaning in the fall. That's when I clean walls, ceilings, windows and closets—everything we used to do in the fall and spring when I was a kid. My family had a very small house compared to the one I live in now. In fact, it takes from October until April to complete the task. As we were expecting guests, I had started the cleaning early, anticipating that I would have about half of the house done before their arrival. I was very tired. It's funny when you are tired and you know that your eyes tell the world of your exhaustion. You know you look bad without even looking in the mirror.

On Wednesday, I had a sore throat. On Thursday, I developed a cough. As I had had that broken rib from coughing two years earlier, I was worried that coughing might re-break the same rib, or any other rib for that matter. I was also worried about what sickness might do to the diabetes. There was a class in the diabetes program dealing with sick days for diabetics, and I wasn't sure that I had paid enough attention to the lessons to be learned.

Anyway, I took precautions. In spite of my reluctance to take any kind of medicine, I decided that perhaps I should take something for the cough. If I had not been diagnosed with diabetes, I would have relied on Werthers to sooth the throat. When I was a kid my mother treated a sore throat with softened butter mixed with sugar to be eaten slowly from a spoon. Guess that treatment was out. On Friday, as I was doing my usual grocery shopping, I stopped at the drug counter to ask the pharmacist for a cough medicine that was suitable for diabetics. I also expressed my concern that I didn't want anything with an antihistamine in it. The only time I had been persuaded to take an antihistamine, I fell asleep watching my pulse jump out of my wrist. The pharmacist assured me that the medicine she gave me was both safe for diabetics and contained no antihistamines.

During the late evening and night, I took the cough medicine as prescribed and slept in a sitting up position to avoid filling up with phlegm. When I woke in the morning, I promised myself the weekend off and jumped out of bed, hurried down the stairs, started pouring the water into the coffee-maker and then—things were "moving" is the only way I can describe it. I put down the water jug and began to call my husband who was in the living room. I have since asked my son what dumb questions he has asked me recently. "What?"

he asked.   "How about: What are you doing down there, Mom?"

At that point I came around to hear his voice. "What are you doing down there, Mom." I was lying on the kitchen floor. As I came to, I started vomiting. I knew enough to ask my son to get my blood glucose testing kit from my office desk downstairs, but when he returned with it, it was soon obvious that I was unable to sit up without getting dizzy all over again. As I pondered whether I should ask him to get me some orange juice, just in case this was a hypoglycemic attack, my son said, "I'm calling 911."

When the paramedics from the fire department arrived, my son kept saying: "My Mom's diabetic, please don't give her any glucose." The medics checked my blood glucose which was neither too low nor too high. They took my vitals, put in an IV port, and held a plastic bag to catch the yellow iridescent vomit which seemed to be nothing but bile and phlegm. When the ambulance arrived, I was carried down the stairs on a stretcher chair and then moved to an ambulance stretcher in the street and lifted into the ambulance. I was amazingly calm.

When we arrived at the hospital, the nurses and the ER doctor took over. They asked everything about my prior medical history. There were many reasons for me to be concerned. There was the old heart arrhythmia, the diabetes with its hypoglycemic and hyperglycemic possibilities. The hospital personnel took my vitals, hooked up a heart monitor, added a blood pressure cuff that self-started at intermittent intervals, took a chest X-ray, followed with a CT scan, and did a urine check.

At one point, one nurse came into the room and remarked with a chuckle: "Oh, you had a full vagal." Both my son and I thought she had said: "Oh, you had a full bagel." We both wondered what she meant. They certainly hadn't fed me in the ER. I said to my son" "If I had a full bagel, I certainly didn't get the cream cheese."

Another nurse thought that I might have had an attack

of Vertigo and I agreed to take a pill for that. What was of concern was that I was still dizzy and unable to get to the bathroom alone. The ER doctor finally said that he thought it might be viral. Then I heard the best news I could have heard. I could hear him on the telephone speaking to someone who turned out to be the doctor they had called in. "Well," he said. "She's a very healthy 64-year-old. I know that she goes to the gym three times a week." I didn't remember telling him I went to the gym, but I wanted to get up and correct him: "More like six or seven times a week."

The doctor who had been called in arrived and checked all of the tests and scans and X-rays. Like everyone else, he wanted to know if I had banged my head in the fall. Another unanswerable question. How would I know that? It was now about 4:00 p.m., and I had been in that room since 6:00 a.m. My son mentioned that he had sat in that room on numerous occasions watching a prisoner chained to that very bed. Just as I thought, things could always be worse. At least I wasn't chained to the bed. From time to time, my son left me for a while. Each time he came back, he said that he had been outside smoking. When I asked who else was out there, he replied that he had been smoking with some of the nurses!

When the doctor said that he wanted to keep me in overnight for observation, I think he expected a protest, but I didn't argue. He was a very nice physician with a good sense of humor. He was very thorough but not an alarmist. He knew my position on drugs—only if absolutely necessary. When he arrived the next day, he said that the only thing that showed anywhere was a chronic condition in the sinuses. At that point, I was able to confirm that I had banged my head in the fall. As I tried to sleep on my back, I soon realized that my head had taken quite a beating. The doctor began to rub his hands over my head, and I soon asked him to stop as that made me dizzy again.

That vasovagal—without cream cheese, provided an opportunity to check out everything except the cholesterol and the Hemoglobin A1c. I did ask one of the nurses if the blood work they had sent to the lab would have shown the cholesterol levels. She did check, but it did not. I would still have to wait a little longer for that.

As I was preparing to leave the hospital, all I could think of was: What if I had ended up in the hospital six months earlier. They would have discovered the undiagnosed diabetes, the cholesterol would have been dangerously high, and the blood pressure would have been in an unacceptable range. Besides all of that, I kept thinking about the paramedics lifting me down that curved staircase on an ambulance chair. What a load of weight I had taken off my mind, my body, and their backs. I also wondered how long I would have been in the hospital if I had presented in my overweight, out-of-shape condition. How many drugs would they have prescribed? The doctor discharged me without any drugs, not even an antibiotic. The work of the last five months had been worth it. Every missed candy bar, every hour at the gym, and all that blood glucose testing. Cliché or not, the diagnosis of diabetes was a blessing in disguise.

~ 12 ~

THE MOMENT OF TRUTH

The bitter and the sweet come from the outside,
the hard from within, from one's own efforts.
                                        ALBERT EINSTEIN

It was October, and the moment of truth was upon me. My doctor and I had agreed that because of the two to three months that it takes to wash the sticky sugar soaked blood from the system, we would wait six months to repeat the Hemoglobin A1c. This would give me three months to replenish the old blood and then give me three months to store up numbers for a new three month average. I was very nervous. I had heard many times that the rotating blood glucose numbers that I was getting from my own testing were just snapshots, not the big picture.

Questions kept going through my mind. Was it possible that I had a faulty meter? Did I misunderstand how to do the test? Was I taking the sample at the wrong time? Was I in some rare class of diabetics whose numbers ran high or low at strange times of the day? In short, were the promising results I had been getting with self-testing close to those we would get with the Hemoglobin A1c? Only the Hemoglobin A1c would give an accurate number for the average of the blood glucose for the last three months.

In the meantime, my blood glucose numbers from 7/9/05 through 10/13/05 were as follows reading left to right:

7/9/05	110	7/10/05	101	7/11/05	92
7/12/05	117	7/13/05	111	7/14/05	100
7/15/05	96	7/16/05	125	7/17/05	104
7/18/05	108	7/19/05	109	7/20/05	104
7/21/05	146	7/22/05	103	7/23/05	88
7/24/05	123	7/25/05	126	7/26/05	109
7/27/05	107	7/28/05	101	7/29/05	89
7/30/05	109	7/31/05	92	8/1/05	105
8/2/05	108	8/3/05	104	8/4/05	92
8/5/05	136	8/6/05	111	8/7/05	110
8/8/05	93	8/9/05	103	8/10/05	107
8/11/05	106	8/12/05	105	8/13/05	101
8/14/05	108	8/15/05	102	8/16/00	94
8/17/05	107	8/18/05	114	8/19/05	107
8/20/05	101	8/21/05	102	8/22/05	110
8/23/05	115	8/24/05	85	8/25/05	112
8/26/05	105	8/27/05	104	8/28/05	94
8/29/05	132	8/30/05	93	8/31/05	102
9/1/05	108	9/2/05	123	9/3/05	150
9/4/05	110	9/5/05	85	9/6/05	128
9/7/05	105	9/8/05	124	9/9/05	117
9/10/05	0	9/11/05	130	9/12/05	101
9/13/05	116	9/14/05	105	9/15/05	113
9/16/05	95	9/17/05	119	9/18/05	96
9/19/05	153	9/20/05	107	9/21/05	112
9/22/05	104	9/23/05	110	9/24/05	149
9/25/05	121	9/26/05	95	9/27/05	115
9/28/05	88	9/29/05	105	9/30/05	96
10/1/05	122	10/2/05	115	10/3/05	108
10/4/05	117	10/5/05	108	10/6/05	95
10/7/05	105	10/8/05	99	10/9/06	139
10/10/05	115	10/11/05	102	10/12/05	93
10/13/05	132				

Here are the 14-day and 30-day averages:

	14 Day Average	30 Day Average
7/9/05 - 7/22/05	109	108
7/23/05 - 8/5/05	106	107
8/6/05 - 8/19/05	105	107
8/20/05 - 9/3/05	110	108
9/4/05 - 9/18/05	110	110
(One extra day added, none recorded on 9/10/05, in the ER that day!)		
9/19/05 - 10/3/05	111	112
10/4/05 - 10/13/05	N/A	N/A
(Only 10 days)		

Here are the high and low numbers for the 14-day periods:

	High	Low
7/9/05 - 7/22/05	146	92
7/23/05 - 8/5/05	136	88
8/6/05 - 8/19/05	114	93
8/20/05 - 9/3/05	150	85
9/4/05 - 9/18/05	130	95
(One extra day added, none recorded on 9/10/05, in the ER that day!)		
9/19/05 - 10/3/05	149	88
10/4/05 - 10/13/05		
(Only 10 days)		

The blood was drawn on 10/13/05. My appointment with the doctor to go over the results was for 10/20/05. When I arrived at the office for the results, the nurse took me into the small office. I asked if my blood tests were back in the file. No, they were not. Now I was becoming agitated. The nurse left to look for the report, but she did not return. Please don't tell me the report was lost or not back yet. I waited for what

seemed like a very long time. Then the doctor tapped lightly
on the door and entered. "Oh, my goodness," she said. "What?
What? What is the Hemoglobin A1c?" "Wow," she said. She
gave me a hug then sat down at the desk. "Look at these numbers." Here they are. She spread out on the desk the first
report and the second report and compared the readings. They
were as follows:

	10/13/05	3/28/05	3/18/05
Hemoglobin A1c			
Hemoglobin A1c	5.7	12.9	
Mean Blood Glucose	114.6	342.8	
Glucose			389
Lipid Panel			
Cholesterol	191		302
Triglycerides	88		282
HDL	52		30
vLDL	17.6		56.4
cLDL	121.4		215.6
Chol/HDL Ratio	3.7		10.1
LDL/HDL Ratio	2.3		7.2

The doctor was excited. "They say you can't reduce
cholesterol levels that much with diet and exercise alone. Just
look at these numbers." Well, I joked, you told me not to come
back until I had lost seventy-five pounds, until my
Hemoglobin A1c was under 6, until my blood pressure was
consistently under 130/80, until my good cholesterol was
raised and until the bad cholesterol was reduced. By the way,
I have now lost 82 lbs." She was soon telling one of the physician's assistants about the results. "You make me feel like a
couch potato," he said to me. "Do you want me to come in and
whip the doctor's into shape?" I laughed.

"It was a good day." I said to the doctor: "You told me
I had to open up my mind to drugs, did you open yours up to
diet and exercise?" "I did," she said. "In fact, there are patients

with whom I would like to share your story, but I am restricted from doing so by the HIPPA laws." She asked if she could
share my first and second blood tests with patients if she took
my name off the sheets. I told her she was welcome to share
my information and my name and my telephone number.
More woman to woman than doctor to patient, she commented: "By the way, you look terrific."

I didn't bother to tell the doctor that my nails were
growing strong and hard. That they were no longer brittle,
breaking, flaking and splitting. I didn't tell her that the
headaches that plagued me for thirty years had finally left. I
still have one cup of regular coffee in the morning but it is not
in reaction to a morning headache. When you wake up
between 4:00 a.m. and 6:00 a.m., there is plenty of time to have
that cup of coffee (without sugar but with milk) and read the
newspaper before eating breakfast at 8:00 a.m. I didn't tell her
that the symptoms from the sciatic hip have left. At one point,
I was walking with a cane while trekking up steep hills in the
villages in the English countryside. No cane needed now. I
didn't tell her that I no longer had acid reflux—don't think I
ever told her about that in the first place. I didn't tell her that
I no longer had to get home in a hurry from the diner because
I no longer have immediate diarrhea. How much of my medical history did the doctor need to hear. She and I had both
heard all we needed to hear for one day.

I did mention that things were not too good at home.
She mentioned that we might need a psychiatrist to do another evaluation. We didn't mention the "S" word. The word I had
said in tears on the day she had called with the diagnosis. The
"S" word—STRESS. "I am under so much stress," I had said.
But she knew that. I wondered back then, if the stress had
brought on the diabetes, and I wondered if I had the strength
and will-power to follow the diet and exercise regime to which
I had committed. I did find the strength to follow the program
and the results were amazing. But, the stress was still there,
sometimes out in the daylight, at other times lurking in the

shadows. What I didn't know was that that stress would be exacerbated and test my coping skills on this quest for health far sooner than I expected.

Part V

Dealing with Stress

~ 13 ~

STRESS TEST

Years steal
Fire from the mind as vigour from the limb;
And Life's enchanted cup but sparkles near the
brim.

LORD BYRON

The nurse who was part of the diabetes workshop asked about stress in my life. She wanted to know what caused the MOST stress and what I did about the stress. During the summer, I participated in a research study being undertaken by the Veterans Administration Memory Clinic in Albany. That study involved engaging in a telephone conference once a week for ten weeks. The Dementia Care Manager worked with women whose husbands had moderate to severe dementia. She worked to help the caregivers deal with both taking care of their husbands who had dementia and with ways to care for themselves while dealing with very stressful situations.

Looking back, I think that when I participated in the Veterans Administration study, I was in denial about how advanced my husband's disease was. At the time, I thought the worst part was dealing with his outbursts and temper-tantrums. During the program, each of the women was asked how they handled the stress of being a caregiver. First of all, I didn't consider myself a caregiver. That, to me, is someone who has to take care of someone else's hygiene needs and there were women in the group who were in that unenviable position.

Even though I knew there were other women with worse situations at home, the Dementia Care Manager wanted to know from me: What do you do to relieve the stress? Go to the gym, I'd replied. That was becoming my mantra: Go to the gym. On a particularly bad week, I had said that I was thinking of going to a hotel for a weekend. What did the other women think about that, she asked. They all thought it was a good idea. A very good idea. Just another fantasy. Of course, I didn't go to the hotel.

To answer the nurse's question during the diabetes workshop, obviously the thing that causes the most stress is my husband's condition. Again, I remembered saying to the doctor when she called with the diagnosis of diabetes: "I have so much stress going on." Now there was the added stress of diabetes and the stress (or reward) of trying to control that diabetes. Dementia and diabetes competing for attention.

"Dementia" was not a word that came easily to my tongue. When my husband was diagnosed in 2001, he was mostly forgetting names, getting confused about things. As an attorney and his partner, I knew that I had to close the office as soon as there was medical confirmation that something serious was happening to him mentally. At that time he had a CT scan that showed moderate shrinkage (atrophy) of the brain. At first, if I was asked why we closed the practice, I'd say that he wasn't as sharp as he used to be. Then, I began to say that he had memory problems. This week, I am finally able to get my mind and my mouth around the dementia word.

During the six months that I was working on turning around the diabetes, things began to exacerbate with my husband's condition. In speaking to our son, he began to refer to me as the woman who lives upstairs, or as the woman who works in the office downstairs. His morning delusions increased and he was often getting dressed at one or two or three in the morning to take a class, or to go to the bank, or to go over the river to that place where they want to sell you something. On the day that I was unconscious on the kitchen floor at 5:30 in the morning, he went into our son's room and said to him: "The woman who lives upstairs is having an attack on the kitchen floor." Thinking it was a "morning moment," my son asked "What are you talking about?"

One night in the winter of 2003, my husband called my name upstairs and said that he thought that there was a mouse in the living room. We had lived in the same house since 1973, and we had never had a mouse in the kitchen on the second floor, just an occasional one in the basement which used to be my formal office before I moved up to the vacated first floor. I got up, got dressed, and went to the local supermarket to buy glue traps and the old-fashioned cheese traps. Neither of us could set the cheese traps, so I left my husband in the living room with about ten sticky pads and the door closed—with a one inch gap at the bottom! The traps were empty the next morning. That night he called upstairs again and said that a mouse had run behind the refrigerator. The following morning, I asked him how sure he was that he had seen a mouse. On a scale of one-ten, ten being sure there was a mouse, how sure was he? A five.

The next day, I called the doctor and asked her if this could be part of the disease. "Yes," she said. "And we do have medicine for that, but I don't want to give it to him yet." That night, I went into the kitchen after dark, and to my shock and horror, a mouse ran behind the refrigerator. We both needed medicine! It turned out that many of the neighbors were infested with mice for the first time and we all went into the "get rid of the infestation" mode with traps and poison.

In the summer of 2004, we were talking to new neighbors, and the topic of bats came up. As we live on the Mohawk River, bat stories are part of the local folklore. I mentioned that we hadn't had a bat in the house for over fourteen years. That night my husband called up the stairs: "Liz. Liz. There's a bat in the house." Now, what was that? A post-hypnotic suggestion manifesting itself in an after-dream state? Or a bat in the house? I called my son in the middle of the night, and he came over from his girlfriend's house and sat with his father in the living room. No bat appeared. As a precaution, we went to the store and spent about twenty minutes picking out a suitable tennis racket as a weapon of choice in case the bat came back. I suppose you could call it the bat to bat the bat with. I called the bat-man and he said that we needed to have the house bat-proofed for several thousand dollars. Another bat-man said that if the bat didn't appear within six days, we could consider that it had died because it wouldn't have had a food source.

Six days after the mysterious bat event, I decided to take a nap. It had been a very sleepless, well-lit series of nights in which any slight sound woke me. While I was taking the nap, my husband called up the stairs. "The bat's back." "Then kill it," I hollered back. He did. Got it with the tennis racket.

Reflecting back now, I realize that even in 2003, my son and I were trying to separate fantasy from reality, to evaluate whether the disease was progressing quickly, to know whether we were in denial as people were telling me that we were. Certainly, we had to acknowledge that the conversations we had with my husband in the mornings were strange. If we could just tell him that he had been dreaming and that there was nowhere that he had to go, that would have been easy. And that's the way it was in the beginning. But now, he wanted to argue, make the dream or delusion a reality, sometimes carrying on the conversation about where he had to go through breakfast and even later.

As our primary physician had suggested an evaluation by a psychiatrist, I called the Veterans Administration. The same Dementia Care Manager with whom I had contact in the support clinic during the summer, set up an appointment for a complete re-evaluation. On November 14, 2005, we went to the Veterans Administration hospital. The physician in charge of the memory clinic was a very adept interviewer. He would put a lot of lawyers to shame with his interrogation techniques. He determined that my husband didn't know, among other things, who the president was, what the year was, what years he was in the military or what years he was in college. When he was asked how many children we have, he said we had two boys. "What are their names?" "I haven't got a clue." The doctor looked at me, my cue to fill in the blanks. "Actually, I said, we have one son." My husband looked surprised: "We do," he said. "I always thought that you had two boys." When I mentioned the fact that he had fallen in the bathtub the week before, my husband said: "That's right, the people who own the property didn't put in a rubber mat." The doctor caught that. "Do you rent your property?" My husband replied: "I don't know." He turned to me and asked: "Who owns that property?" "We do," I replied.

There was a lot more yet to be revealed in the long evaluation which appeared to be directed more towards informing me as the caregiver than towards my husband the patient. If I had been in a state of denial, that denial was being stripped away layer by layer. There was still fire in my husband's mind but it was no longer directed towards the opposition in a legal trial. Now it was being fanned by ghosts of the past who were feeding him inaccurate information. I was overwhelmed with sadness, fear and responsibility.

~ 14 ~

STAYING WITH THE PROGRAM

All work of man is as the swimmer's: a waste
[vast] ocean threatens to devour him; if he front
it not bravely, it will keep its word.

THOMAS CARLYLE

Towards the end of the meeting with the doctor at the Veterans Administration, he looked over the four-year-old CT scan and pointed out that there were strokes on the film. I hadn't known that. He pointed out what I did know that there was moderate cortical atrophy. He said that the condition was very advanced and that I should join a support group. At that point the Dementia Care Manager was in the doorway. "The gym," she said. "Keep going to the gym."

It had been a long day. I hadn't slept the night before worrying about what we would learn. And I knew I would lose another night's sleep worrying about what we did learn. The doctor asked my husband if he was incontinent. My husband replied that he was not. The doctor then said that he didn't know why my husband wasn't incontinent and why he wasn't having motor problems. And he commented that those observations were being made on a CT scan that was over four years old. The doctor gave the alcohol and smoking lecture, which fell on deaf ears, just as the high blood pressure, high cholesterol, and being overweight lecture hadn't scared me into action. The doctor talked about the lack of oxygen to the brain. He wanted to do another CT scan, but there was no cooperation on that. In fact, I was surprised that he had managed to keep my husband there for as long as he did.

The good news was that he wasn't incontinent. He didn't have motor problems. But were those things to expect in the near future? Were they things to worry about now or later? Very advanced. The words kept ringing in my mind. Very advanced. And I never asked the questions I wanted answered. How fast would this progress? Could he stay at this level for a few years? I think I knew that there really were no answers to those questions.

The doctor remarked several times that my husband was an independent thinker. I think one time he said that was one of the times when my husband put on his coat and said he was leaving. The doctor had got all he was getting of him. He had been flashing dirty looks my way after about the first ten minutes of the lengthy session. He is fiercely independent. He is the ultimate illustration of Carpe Diem, Seize the Day. But now as I watched this evaluation unfold, I knew that my husband's independence was being devoured by dementia. What a state of denial I had been in.

So, here I was with more questions than I had answers. It was a long drive over to Albany and the traffic was very bad on the way home. Exhausted from no sleep and with my brain in overdrive, I was ready to make dinner and head for bed. But then I caught myself. Some drink, some use drugs, and some eat to relieve stress. I had been a stress eater. This time, it didn't occur to me to eat, but I was thinking about not going to the gym for a second day in a row. My 14-day chart for blood pressure and blood glucose readings now includes a check mark when I attend the gym. My doctor had said at the "good news" meeting that it was all right to take a day off from the gym once in a while. My bargain with myself was that I needed at least five, preferably seven, red ticks before I miss a day at the gym. Unless I am sick, I do not miss two days in a row. I had had seven ticks before I missed the first day, the day before we went to the Veterans Administration hospital, but now I was considering a second day off in a row.

I heard the words of the nurse in the diabetes program reverberating in my brain. Go to the gym every day. I heard the words of the Dementia Care Manager from the Veterans Administration as she stood in the doorway as the doctor was delivering the bad news. Go to the gym. Go to the gym. I heard the words of my own doctor. Go to the gym. Did the Dementia Care Manager know that the news that day might be an upset to my good work. When she had said "go to the gym" as we were leaving the doctor's office, I said: "Eighty-five pounds. I have lost eighty-five pounds." She turned to the doctor. "Elizabeth turned her diabetes around." "And the cholesterol, and the blood pressure," I added. "You did?" he asked, then pondered aloud: "It's all about our lifestyles and the choices we make."

With the words of all those professionals ringing in my ears, I checked to make sure my son would be in the house for an hour or so, then I put on my sneakers and headed out of the door. When I got back home from the gym, I made dinner and went to bed early. It was time for more reflection. How long would it take for me to be back in the obese category and have a Hemoglobin A1c in the 12.9 range again if I let my own healthcare slip now. I had toyed with defeat when I had considered missing the gym for a second day. What would I do when things got worse with the dementia? And it seemed that worse was what we were to expect, sooner than I had anticipated. Would I revert to my old habit of stress eating? Would I forget about portion control, add back a candy-bar or a bowl of ice-cream? Would I find a reason not to go to the gym—too tired, too busy, too much stress?

There is a guilt aspect in taking care of myself. I have always known that if someone around me has a problem, then

taking care of myself seems like a selfish act. It was in a Weight
Watchers® meeting that I made that observation. I had asked:
"How can I justify taking care of myself if someone around me
has a worse problem than being overweight?" As if being overweight wasn't a real problem. Maybe at that time I didn't
understand how serious being overweight can be. In response
to my statement, another member commented: "But if you
don't take care of yourself, how can you take care of others?" I
wasn't convinced of that at that time, but knowing what I now
knew about diabetes and dementia, that comment seemed to
make sense. Taking care of my own health as well as the health
of my husband was something I must not lose sight of—unless
I was willing to let that vast ocean of stress devour me.

~ 15 ~

"It's All About Me"

How sickness enlarges the dimensions of a man's self to himself! he is his own exclusive object. Supreme selfishness is inculcated upon him as his only duty.

CHARLES LAMB

Something had been bothering me about my reflection that if I didn't take care of myself, I couldn't take care of others. What was bothering me was hard to put my finger on. It was just a few days after our visit to the Veterans Administration that I spoke on the telephone with the Diabetes Program Coordinator at Ellis Hospital in Schenectady. She described a program being offered at the hospital to hospital staff at risk for developing type 2 diabetes. She explained the program and said that the title was "It's All About Me." The program was being funded partially by a grant awarded by the New York State Health Department and the Capital District Coalition for Diabetes Prevention.

After talking about the program designed to help with the prevention of diabetes and my experience in treating the disease, the Diabetes Program Coordinator asked if I would like to speak in one of their classes taking place in December. I readily accepted. She said she would give the main lecture and asked if I would speak for fifteen minutes. That was easy.

After I hung up the telephone, I immediately began to ponder what inspirational message I might impart to people at risk for the development of diabetes, an audience which included many nurses. When I had thought about becoming involved in diabetes education, I had prepared a list of targeted audiences. That list included the following people and organizations, in the following order:

TARGET AUDIENCES

1) Newly diagnosed patients who are trying to avoid oral drugs and/or insulin treatment and who seek an alternative method of blood glucose control.

2) Patients who are on drugs and/or insulin therapy and seek ways to improve the condition of diabetes and reduce or eliminate dependence on drugs and/or insulin.

3) Physicians in the diabetes field who are trained in the medical model but who also are open-minded to alternative methods of controlling diabetes.

4) HMOs who stand to gain from educating patients and avoiding the cost of drugs, insulin, and the very expensive medical treatment associated with the complications of uncontrolled diabetes.

5) The American Diabetes Association and The American Dietetic Association, the leading educators for people with diabetes and who are best equipped to reach those millions of people who are willing to consider a non-medical model to control diabetes.

6) AARP, whose members seek alternatives to traditional medicine and who are seeking to live long and healthy lives.

7) State Health Departments charged with the education of their residents on health issues.

8) Federal Health Officials who are charged with the education of all of the people with, or at risk for, diabetes in the U.S.

9) Anyone identified as being in a high risk group, such as those who are overweight or who are said to have a genetic pre-disposition to the disease.

10) Anyone who wants to lose weight, control blood pressure or improve cholesterol levels with the added benefit of reducing the risk of developing diabetes.

The group to whom I would be addressing my comments fell at the bottom of my targeted audience list. Perhaps I had the list in the wrong order. What better place to start than with prevention.

As I thought about my short talk, I knew that I could relate to the audience by talking about my own exercise and diet program. I could also talk about what that exercise entailed and what, when, and how much I ate. I could talk about my own success in controlling diabetes, reworking cholesterol levels, regulating blood pressure and reducing weight—the total health makeover. I could read the numbers from my laboratory test reports as confirmation of the fact that the effort is really worthwhile. I could talk about the role of stress in developing disease and the need to stay protected from that stress as we address our health needs.

The Coordinator had mentioned that twenty-four Ellis Hospital employees had signed up for the program. They were all women. Not one man had taken advantage of the opportunity to learn more about the prevention of diabetes. As she pointed out, men have women to take care of them. Women are the nurturers. They take care of others, she reflected, but do they take care of themselves? She mentioned that the local newspaper, *The Daily Gazette*, was publishing an article on the program the next day.

As I continued to ponder on the focus of my short talk, I was still having this niggling thought that something was wrong with my earlier statement about taking care of myself to be able to take care of others. As I read the article in *The Daily Gazette* dated November 22, 2005, and entitled "It's all about diabetes," I was struck by the comment of one of the participants in the program. She was quoted as saying: "I think women struggle more with 'move more, eat less,' because they are often busy taking care of everyone else but themselves. . . . But if you're healthy, you'll be better able to take care of others."

That was what had been bothering me—the notion that we take care of ourselves in order to take care of others. In the article in *The Daily Gazette*, Joanne DiNovio, Certified Diabetes Educator and Program Coordinator for The Ellis Hospital Center for Diabetes, was quoted as saying: "[T]he 'me' in 'It's All About Me' stands for 'move more, eat less.'" She added: "We decided to incorporate the 'me' factor because I think that 'eat less, move more' doesn't always work if the person hasn't made a commitment . . . so part of the curriculum is going to be making the decision to care for yourself."

That was the missing piece for my talk and answered my own question. I would tell the audience that they did need to move more and eat less, a concept that I had incorporated into my own wellness plan. But I would also tell them that they knew something that I was still working on—the need to take care of ourselves for our own sakes, not just for the sake of others. We don't need permission to do the same for our-selves as we do for our loved ones. ME is a little two-letter word that has importance and significance for all of us. No permission needed. No martyr complexes here. I had my short talk in the bag, and I had taken something from the pro-gram for myself.

The morning delusions took on new importance on the day I was to give this talk at the hospital. It was 3:00 a.m. when I was awakened by a loud noise in the house. Sitting up in bed, I tried to figure out what the noise was when the burglar alarm started its shrill sound. By the time I made it down one flight of stairs, the telephone was ringing. It was the alarm company service operator calling to see if we needed assistance. I wasn't sure if my husband had tripped the alarm and was downstairs trying to figure out how to turn it back off. Looking down the stairs, I could see no sign of him. I asked the operator to hold while I checked the living room. He wasn't there, either. I asked the operator to hold again while I went downstairs to turn off the alarm. When I got back upstairs to the telephone, I explained to her that my husband seemed to have wandered from the house. She asked if she should send the police to help look for my husband. That would be a good idea. But as she put me on hold, there was pounding on the front door.

While the operator was calling the police, I put the tele-phone down and went downstairs and opened the front door. At the front door was my husband with his hair all disheveled and with blood on his face across the bridge of the nose. The car was running outside of the house. "Come on," he said. "You have to come with me to Amsterdam to pick up the other car. I've asked everyone else, and no-one would come with me." I asked: "What happened to your face?" He replied: "Something fell off the dashboard and hit me." Later, he said: "I hit the brake too hard and hit my head." He was acting out one of his morning delusions, but this was the first time he had headed out of the house. As I mentioned earlier, either my son or I usually hear him moving around and putting on his coat and one of us persuades him that he had been dreaming and that there was nowhere he needed to go. Now there were new issues with driving and safety—his, mine and others. When I suggested that I should take the keys at night, he became very belligerent. More stress on the horizon.

I shared the story with the women in the at-risk for diabetes group to illustrate the importance of recognizing and dealing with stress. The dietician from that program said to me afterwards. "And you came here today, after that?" Absolutely. I also worked in my office all day and went to the gym. As abnormal becomes the norm, I am learning to adjust. When my husband asks where the boys are, I respond that I don't know. Tongue in cheek, I mentioned to our son—one of them—that I might become part of a folie à deux (a delusional system shared by two people who share a close relationship).

As I was invited as a motivational speaker, I said in conclusion that perhaps I needed to be more motivated to stay with the plan than they did because I was now diabetic. On the other hand, maybe they needed to be more motivated than I was in order never to have to say: "Hi, my name is (Mary), and I'm a diabetic."

Part VI

Refining the Eating Plan

~ 16 ~

POTATOES, ANYONE?

*Sweet potatoes or yams are lower on the GI scale
and thus should be preferred over white potatoes.*
RICHARD N. PODELL, M.D., F.A.C.P.

There were certain starches that I had been thinking about as possibilities to add back into my diet and include on my list of acceptable foods. Potatoes were of particular interest and concern. For over eight months, I had left potatoes out of my diet completely. Certainly, the diet in my last life had contained many potatoes, baked, fried, mashed, roasted and boiled. Anyone on a serious diet knows that the french fries need to go, if not for the starch element, at least for the fat. But now I had learned that baked and mashed potatoes were particularly high on the Glycemic Index, so I was done with them.

The question I was asking myself was whether or not to include boiled potatoes and/or sweet potatoes or yams. Baked and mashed potatoes come in at the same high number on the Glycemic Index as one teaspoon of table sugar. Boiled potatoes are higher than sweet potatoes or yams (Podell, 1993, 62). One evening, as I was making one of my family's favorite dishes of poached salmon with mayonnaise sauce, I decided this would be a perfect opportunity to try boiled potatoes. It was an evening during which the blood glucose was to be taken two hours after dinner. The salmon was prepared in a Turbo-Cooker, one of my favorite cooking pots. On the bottom of the pot, I poured in small canned boiled potatoes, washed well first to remove any starch that had leeched into the water. About a cup of fresh clean water was added to the potatoes. The salmon was placed on the grill above the potatoes and water. On went the lid, and the salmon was poached. When I cooked this dish for my family before the diagnosis of diabetes, once the salmon was poached, I added butter to the potatoes in the bottom of the pan. Well, the butter had to go. Perhaps olive oil would work as well.

The olive oil browned the potatoes nicely. When the dish was completed, I placed two servings of salmon on two plates, drizzled over the mayonnaise sauce, measured out the potatoes to equal 30 grams of carbohydrates for me, and added Brussels sprouts to my plate. As I put a piece of potato in my mouth, my head took over. I had been saying for a long time that the control was now in my head, not in my mouth. This experiment didn't feel right. I took the first bite, afraid that I would fall in love with potatoes again after not tasting them for over eight months. Then a strange thing happened. First of all, the taste wasn't nearly as good as I had expected. Perhaps it was because I had used olive oil in place of butter. I didn't think so. There was something more important taking place here. I couldn't swallow the potato in my mouth. My head was working overtime, thinking about the blood glucose test that was to take place later and the good average I was main-taining at the moment. I spat the potato out. If I had had time, I would have prepared coucous or a pasta product, but I used my stand-by favorite—three whole grain Wasa® crackers spread with Benecol® Light.

Those of you paying attention probably know that Podell's Glycemic Index rating for Wasa® crackers is the same as that for boiled potatoes (1993, 284.) Well, I knew one thing for certain, my readings were always good with the crackers, and I wasn't ready to take a chance on the potatoes. Maybe I could eat them without wrecking by blood glucose averages, but it wasn't that important. My dinner was delicious, tasted even better for the control that I had discovered was now part of my soul. If a potato didn't make it past my mouth and into my stomach, what chance did a candy-bar have? Two hours later, I tested my blood—95!

Next came the yams or sweet potatoes. Actually, I had tried sweet potatoes on one occasion. It was Thanksgiving, and we had walked up to the restaurant just one block from home. I had been prepared. In my pocketbook, just in case— you guessed it—were three Wasa® crackers in a zip-lock bag. The buffet was spectacular and filled with luscious desserts no longer on my diet. Actually, there was only one concern for me. It wasn't that I couldn't eat the pastries, but whether they offered anything in the starch group besides mashed potatoes. Only sweet potatoes. But why were they shiny? Were they covered in maple syrup?

As I approached the carving station and asked for a very small slice of ham and an even smaller slice of turkey, I asked the carver if there was syrup on the sweet potatoes. She confirmed that there was and asked if she could help me with something. I said that it was all right, but I would have liked a starch other than mashed potatoes or sweet potatoes covered in maple syrup.

As I moved away to serve green beans on my plate, I saw the carver head towards the kitchen and out came the chef. The chef at this restaurant had owned another one in town which my husband and I had frequented very often. He was very obliging and offered to make anything I wanted. Just a small plate of plain pasta would be great.

When the waitress came to the table she said: "Doug said he didn't recognize you at first because you had lost so much weight. He said when he saw who it was, you could have anything you wanted. Here's some pasta. He also said that he had heard that you would like sweet potatoes without maple syrup, and here is a plate of those, also."

I ate some of the sweet potatoes and some of the pasta. Actually, I didn't dislike the sweet potatoes. They were new to me when I came here from England in the late 1960s. I thought they were disgusting. When I asked the waitress if sweet potatoes used to have marshmallows on them, she said, "Yamallos. They used to call them yamallos. Sweet potatoes with maple syrup and small marshmallows on top." No wonder I never liked them, but I didn't mind them now. What I needed to do was to try them at home and test to see if, or how much, they spiked the blood glucose. But, first of all, I needed to determine the difference between sweet potatoes and yams.

After a discussion with a very nice man in the produce section at the supermarket, it soon became clear to me why references to sweet potatoes and yams often are lumped in one statement. He showed me a book meant to be useful in identifying vegetables and a general blurb about how to cook them and how they contributed to a healthy diet. When I arrived home, I read some more about sweet potatoes and yams. Suffice it to say that the discussions on sweet potatoes and yams were very interesting but not worth analyzing here. After all, the premise is KEEP IT SIMPLE. From now on I will refer to "sweet potatoes or yams" as others do.

It was easier at home to measure the servings and to eat the sweet potatoes or yams at a meal after which blood glucose testing was scheduled. Two servings equaled about six ounces. They were cut into inch size cubes and boiled until almost tender, then frozen baby Brussels sprouts were added for the last few minutes. Both vegetables were strained and topped with Benecol® Light. It was nice to have the texture of potatoes back in the diet, but I can't say that I was particularly impressed with the taste. Blood Glucose Number—120.

The second time that I tried sweet potatoes was when I ordered a hamburger with Irish fries—fried sweet potatoes or yams served at the restaurant mentioned later in the chapter on *Eating Out and Fast Food*. I'm not sure what the shock of the first deep-fried food to enter my digestive system in almost a year had on my cholesterol levels, but at least I could check on what affect the consumption of sweet potatoes or yams had on the blood glucose. I must admit that those sweet potatoes or yams were far more enticing than the ones I had tried earlier. Blood Glucose Number—111.

Sweet potatoes or yams were now coming into play in my new diet. But what I soon realized about sweet potatoes was that they present the same problem as white potatoes. How would they taste best: deep-fried, baked, mashed, or roasted? We know all about the fat content of deep-frying, to which I had just succumbed with the Irish fries. Baked potatoes are usually topped with some combination of butter, sour cream, bacon bits and cheese. Mashed potatoes come with the usual butter and cream. Roasted in the pan around the meat soaked in the meat drippings wasn't a very good option either. For now, I will use sweet potatoes one of two ways. One is to simply boil them, with or without another vegetable, and top them with a pat of Benecol® Light. The other way? Well, you know what that is. The one deep-fried food now allowed in my diet and available at a local restaurant—but only occasionally, you have my word on that. The more I think about including sweet potatoes or yams into recipes, I wonder whether they could be used in a healthy way. Sounds like a project for the kitchen.

~ 17 ~

MORE STARCH EXPERIMENTS

O do you know the muffin man,
The muffin man, the muffin man,
O do you know the muffin man,
That lives in Drury Lane?

THE MUFFIN MAN
ANONYMOUS

After the experiments with the potatoes, there were more foods on the list to be consumed followed by blood glucose testing. The items which were on the list were starches that had been left out of the diet initially for various reasons. It had been difficult to find whole-wheat muffins without a lot of added sugar. It would take some time to keep looking at the food labels in the bread isle.

One time I tried buckwheat pancakes with blueberries and the blood glucose number had been high. That time I had consumed two servings of starch with the blueberries and the appropriate protein and vegetables for lunch. Would it make a difference to the blood glucose if this item was served at breakfast with only one starch? What about if I left out the blueberries? What if I added the blueberries back in? Although I always included four ounces of orange juice at dinner, since trying blueberry buckwheat pancakes and having a high blood glucose reading, I had always reserved fruit for an afternoon snack rather than including it with a meal.

As regular white and brown rice generally were not recommended on the Glycemic Index, they were eliminated from my diet. Then I read in several sources that Basmati rice was a better choice for keeping blood glucose numbers stable. That was worth a try.

The targeted foods were, then: whole-wheat English Muffins, buckwheat pancakes, and Basmati rice. Nothing scientific here. Just test the blood glucose number after consuming each food three times and record the results. Other diabetics might have a different blood glucose reading after consuming these particular foods. It is hoped that this section will work as inspiration to others to make their own "unscientific" experiments and expand their healthy food choices with confidence.

ENGLISH MUFFINS
Thomas'® Hearty Grains English Muffins

1) Served one half English Muffin spread with Benecol® Light with one egg and 1/2 glass of milk for breakfast.
Blood Glucose Number—86

2) Served one half English Muffin spread with Benecol® Light with one ounce of Cabot's 50% fat-free cheese and 1/2 glass of milk for breakfast.   *Blood Glucose Number—96*

3) Served one half English Muffin spread with one tablespoon of peanut butter and 1/2 glass of milk for breakfast.
Blood Glucose Number—107

BUCKWHEAT PANCAKES
Arrowhead Mills® Buckwheat Pancake & Waffle Mix

1) Made one pancake, one serving, using water only to mix. Other ingredients listed on package were omitted. This was cooked in

a heated frying pan sprayed with Pam® Butter Spray and served with two links of Armor® Brown'N Serve Fully Cooked Turkey Sausage Links and 1/2 glass of milk for breakfast.

Blood Glucose Number—115

2) It was a Saturday morning and I had time to make something a little more time-consuming than my usual oatmeal for breakfast. Actually oatmeal is often the only breakfast that I eat for several days in a row. Anyway, this was a day to test the blood glucose after breakfast, so I decided to try the buckwheat pancakes and to eat three slices of lean bacon. Bacon is on the list of "once-in-a-great-while" foods. Well, there were blueberries in the refrigerator and I decided to try them in the pancake again. Weighing the few berries that I had ready to add to the pancake showed that 1/2 ounce was all that was needed for one blueberry pancake. So, it was one blueberry buckwheat pancake with 3 slices of lean bacon and 1/2 cup of milk.

Blood Glucose Number—92

3) Served one Blueberry Buckwheat Pancake with Benecol® Light and one egg lightly beaten and cooked in a frying pan coated with non-stick butter spray and 1/2 cup of milk.

Blood Glucose Number—82

BASMATI RICE
Della® Gourmet Rice Aromatic American Basmati Brown Rice

1) Cooked just shy of one cup of Basmati rice according to package directions. Sautéed chopped garlic, one cup of chopped mushrooms and one cup of sliced onions in olive oil. Added half of the cooked rice to the frying pan and continued to sauté for a few more minutes. Stirred in four ounces of bite size pieces of poached salmon and served on two plates for lunch. The left over rice was saved for another meal.

Blood Glucose Number—102

2) Cooked Basmati rice was now in containers in the refrigerator waiting for the next opportunity to test the blood glucose after

consuming rice with other foods. One day we were mulling over lunch when my son suggested a Chinese take-out. Very good idea! In the past when we ordered Chinese, I always ordered a pint of vegetable Lo Mein to go with my order and measured out what seemed to be two servings to go with my chicken and broccoli. Looking for something different, I ordered beef and sugar snap peas to serve over two servings of warmed-up Basmati rice. It tasted delicious. What about the blood glucose number?   *Blood Glucose Number—92*

3) It was around midnight when my son arrived home from a trip to the supermarket on his way home from work. He had all the ingredients for Quiche Lorraine and he called me on the telephone by the bed. Is there any way you can eat this, Mom? In a sleepy state, I said I didn't think so, but as I lay there it crossed my mind that maybe a quiche could be made with a rice crust. I was too tired to try to explain this to him at that late hour. The next day, I took eight servings of cooked rice and pressed them into a pie plate pre-sprayed with Pam® Butter Spray. My son asked what I was doing. "How about this for a pie shell?" I asked. "Want me to make that into a quiche?" he responded. The offer was too good to turn down. For dinner, I had one quarter of the quiche (two starch servings and 2 1/2 protein servings) with a salad tossed in olive oil and balsamic vinegar. Delicious. As an aside, the next day my son asked if the quiche had been too rich. For a moment, I thought that he had sneaked cream in and not the regular milk I had agreed to let him use. He didn't think my usual 1% would make it creamy enough. "You used regular milk and not cream?" I asked him. "Oh, yes," he replied, then added, "but I was just wondering about the half a stick of butter." He caught me for a second, but when I looked at his face, he burst out laughing.

Blood Glucose Number—97

~ 18 ~

WEIGHTS AND MEASURES

What is food to one, is to others bitter poison.
LUCRETIUS

Weighing and measuring has become a part of my life since the diagnosis of diabetes, but as well as weighing foods and measuring drinks, I needed to take stock of all of the items that routinely found their way into my kitchen cabinets and into the refrigerator and freezer. A lot of items needed to be tossed, and a lot of items needed to stay on the shelf in the grocery store never to find their way into our house again. On the other hand, my husband is not diabetic and there were foods that he would still want to have available. The trick here was to determine what "junk" foods he wanted and what "junk" foods were in the house just for me. This would take a real honest chat with myself about those foods to which I was addicted and the need to remove them from my kitchen. It would also take a certain degree of control to avoid the foods that were on my husband's list of "staples."

The old "c-items" were a good place to start: chocolate, candy, chips, cookies, cream, coke, cake mixes, cake toppings, cereal (other than oatmeal) and crackers (other than Wasa®). Let's be honest, no-one except me really cared about potato chips and corn chips. They could be tossed and taken off the shopping list. Chocolate, candy, cookies, cream, coke, cake, cereal (sugar-frosted flakes) and white crackers were on my husband's list and they would still need to be brought into the house. The only one of these items which was a favorite of mine was chocolate. Well, I soon got used to seeing a mental picture of bars of Cadbury's Milk Chocolate with a skull and crossbones on them. That was hard for an English girl who grew up close to the Cadbury's chocolate factory.

Besides the cookies and cake mixes to be left in the house for my husband, there were other white flour products—white flour itself used for gravy and baking, croutons and breadcrumbs—all tossed.

Apart from the items on my husband's needs list, all other items were tossed if they contained artificial sweeteners or an added grain of sugar. The bag of sugar stayed in the cupboard for his coffee.

To weigh food, I invested in a lovely silver-colored scale—practical but attractive enough to be on display in the kitchen. One afternoon, I wandered up and down the isles at the store and came home with several one-cup measuring cups, two four-ounce measuring glasses, several sets of measuring spoons and two four-ounce plastic containers. Years ago, we were always looking for THE scissors, and I thought how silly is that. We have three television sets and one pair of scissors. That was when I learned how easy it makes life if you have several often-used items in handy places. I bought six pairs of scissors and left them all over the house. In the same way, measuring cups and measuring spoons all seemed to be in the dishwasher when they were needed. Time to have lots of measuring cups and measuring spoons handy.

Now that I had the weighing and measuring equipment, what did I weigh and measure? Just about all foods and drinks that I consumed. Pasta—weighed. Couscous—weighed. Cheese—weighed. Meat—weighed. Oatmeal—measured. Milk—measured. Orange Juice—measured. Vegetables—often a rough measure. Fruit—sometimes weighed. Fat—measured at first, but not later on after I settled on Benecol Light®, Olive Oil, and Light Mayonnaise—with a small slice of avocado and a small portion of sour cream once in a while.

Portion control was an absolute must in this new plan, and the only way to be sure how much was being consumed was to weigh and measure just about everything going into the diet. I am glad that every item coming out of the supermarket now has nutrition and portion sizes on the labels. That makes checking for protein and carbohydrate content very easy.

In addition to weighing and measuring foods and drinks, I was weighing and measuring other things. I was weighing myself on the bathroom scale. The weight dropped off at about two pounds a week. The good news was that I didn't have to have a discussion with myself about what I had eaten that had caused some of the weight to re-appear. It never did! Sometimes the weight plateaued for a few days, but it never went back up. My belief was that as long as I stayed on the diet—weighing and measuring—my weight would end up where it was meant to be. No more indulging one day and cutting back the next. This was proving to be really easy. Why hadn't I had an appointment with a dietitian years ago. All I had to do was eat well-balanced meals three times a day, watch the portions, and I was shaping up to be a thin lady once again.

Measuring was also a part of my life outside of the kitchen. Measure the glucose in the blood by taking blood samples daily. Measure the blood pressure at the gym. The only thing I couldn't measure was the cholesterol. But with the recent results, I wasn't too concerned about that anymore. My ability to self-monitor my progress and to have a project that was both fun and rewarding was something I enjoyed. I was learning to re-program my brain and put the thinking back in my head and not my mouth—the potato experiment showed that this was working.

I no longer flinched when I saw the commercial. You

know the one that I mean. When diet and exercise are not enough? That's right, another pill—this one for cholesterol. Sometimes I paid attention to the drugs being touted on the commercials on the television. It is strange to be told to ask your doctor about a certain drug without being told what it is for. How ridiculous is that. Do people really go to the doctor's office with a list of pills advertised on the television and ask for a prescription for one or a combination of them? For my part, I was ready to keep on weighing my body and my food, ready to keep on measuring liquids, ready to keep on testing my blood glucose and my blood pressure. Maybe my Aunt Tillie and my Uncle Harry had passed on a gene for diabetes, for high cholesterol, for high blood pressure, or for obesity, but I wasn't worried. Even if they had, it turns out that diet and exercise can be enough. Maybe not for everyone, but certainly for me.

As the weeks passed, my kitchen became a special place. At first my meals were rather simple, but as the months progressed I learned to modify old favorite recipes, create new recipes, and engage in a ritual of combining the right portions of fat, starches, and protein in appetizing meals. Most of the time, I served my husband what I was eating. He might end his meal with a bowl of ice-cream or a piece of cake. Sometimes, I bought him pastries at the new bakery in town. But as the old saying goes: One man's meat is another man's poison. And I knew what was poison to me. Or, more accurately, I knew what foods acted as medicine. What a relief to know that the solution to my problem was in my refrigerator and kitchen cabinets and not in a pill bottle or a hypodermic needle.

Part VII

The What, When and Where of the Diet

~ 19 ~

THE BASIC MODIFIED DAILY DIET

The morning cup of coffee has an exhilaration about it which the cheering influence of the afternoon or evening cup of tea cannot be expected to reproduce.

OLIVER WENDELL HOLMES, SR.

1-2 HOURS BEFORE BREAKFAST
1 cup of coffee
1/2 cup of 1% milk

BREAKFAST
1 starch serving
1 protein serving
1/2 cup of 1% milk <u>or</u> 1/3 cup of low-fat yogurt <u>or</u>
1/2 cup of buttermilk
Fat

BETWEEN BREAKFAST AND LUNCH
1/2 cup of 1% milk <u>or</u> 1/3 cup of low-fat yogurt

LUNCH
2 starch servings
2 protein servings
1 1/2 servings of non-starchy vegetables
Fat

BETWEEN LUNCH AND DINNER
1 Fruit

DINNER
2 starch servings
3 protein servings
1 1/2 servings of non-starchy vegetables
Fat
1/2 cup juice (for me, this is combined with 1 1/2 ounces of gin)

AFTER DINNER
1/2 cup of 1% milk or 1/3 cup of low-fat yogurt

~ 20 ~

BREAKFAST, LUNCH, AND DINNER

Tell me what you eat, and I will tell you who you are.

ANTHELME BRILLAT-SAVARIN

<u>BREAKFAST SERVINGS</u>*
1 starch
1 protein
1 fat
1/2 milk

<u>BREAKFAST SUGGESTIONS</u>
Starches
1 serving of steelcut oatmeal <u>or</u>
1 slice of 100% stoneground whole wheat, sprouted barley,
sprouted rye seed, sprouted sourdough, sprouted wheat,
pumpernickel or rye bread <u>or</u>
1/2 whole grain English muffin <u>or</u>
1 buckweat pancake <u>or</u>
1 1/2 Wasa® crackers

Protein
1 ounce of 50% fat-free cheese <u>or</u>
2 ounces of Ricotta cheese <u>or</u>

1 egg or
1 ounce of Lox or
1 tablespoon of peanut butter or
2 turkey sausages or
3 slices regular lean bacon or
3 slices of canadian bacon

Fat
Benecol Light® spread on bread or stirred into the oatmeal

Milk
1/2 cup of 1% or
1/3 cup of yogurt or
1/2 cup buttermilk

LUNCH AND DINNER SERVINGS*
2 starches
2 protein (lunch) 3 protein (dinner)
1 1/2 servings of non-starchy vegetables
Fat

LUNCH AND DINNER SUGGESTIONS
Starches
2 slices of 100% stoneground whole wheat, sprouted barley,
sprouted rye seed, sprouted sourdough, sprouted wheat,
pumpernickel or rye bread or
2 servings of whole wheat buns or
2 servings of buckwheat groats or
2 servings of bulgur wheat or
3 Wasa® crackers or
2 servings of coucous or
2 servings of kasha or
2 servings of pasta—whole wheat preferred or
2 servings of pita bread or

2 servings of Basmati rice <u>or</u>
4 Taco shells <u>or</u>
2 servings of sweet potatoes or yams

Protein
(2 servings of any combination of the following for lunch and
3 servings of any combination for dinner)
Bacon
Cheese
Eggs
Fish
Meat
Peanut Butter
Poultry
Sausage
Seafood
Tofu

Fat
Avocado <u>or</u>
Benecol® Light Spread <u>or</u>
Light Mayonnaise <u>or</u>
Olive Oil <u>or</u>
Sour Cream

Vegetables
1 1/2 servings of non-starchy vegetables

See the recipes in Chapter 24 for suggestions on combining the
above servings for lunch and dinner.

*For more information on serving sizes, see Chapter 22.

~ 21 ~

EATING OUT AND FAST FOOD

If you have formed the habit of checking on every new diet that comes along, you will find that, mercifully, they all blur together, leaving you with only one definite piece of information: french-fried potatoes are out.

JEAN KERR

For many months after being diagnosed with diabetes, I approached eating out and fast food take-out with trepidation. As I was sitting with my doctor on the day when I received the diabetes diagnosis, one of the staff members called her and asked if she wanted Chinese for lunch. I commented that my days of eating Chinese food were over. She had replied that they were not. I had mumbled that they only serve white rice. Well, eat just a little. What about Jumpin' Jacks, the favorite hamburger place in the summer for locals? You can have the burger, just eat half of the bun.

Jumpin' Jacks was the first treat to make its way into my new diet. With a whole wheat bun in a small plastic bag in my pocket book, I switched rolls at the table. Later, someone told me to just ask for an Atkins burger and add my own roll. I tried the cole slaw as a vegetable, but it was just too salty for my taste. Did I ever mention salt? It is a very rare occasion that I add salt to my food at the table. If I am cooking a dish for other people, I do add salt but in very limited amounts.

Chinese take-out was second on the "put back" list. As I mentioned earlier, once I realized that pasta was acceptable on the Glycemic Index, I ordered chicken broccoli and a pint of vegetable Lo Mein. From the Lo Mein, I measured out what I thought was two servings of starches. Later on, I replaced the Lo Mein with Basmati rice and added beef and sugar snap peas to my acceptable choices of Chinese take-out food. Yes, I do sometimes go the lengths of taking the meat and vegetables apart and measuring and weighing.

Taco Bell was third on the need to function in the "real world" of eating out at fast food places. The choice here was two crispy tacos. That was as close as I could come to making a wise choice. Even though two tacos makes the meal light on starches, just two shells are packed with protein.

Some rules developed for eating out in restaurants:

1) If I am going to have my daily cocktail at that meal, I carry four ounces of fresh-squeezed juice in a small container in my pocket book. Sometimes it is very difficult to communicate with the staff that I need a large glass with space for my own juice. We get it right, eventually. One time when I forgot the juice, I had a beer rather than risk commercial juices. That time, my blood glucose was less than 100, in spite of my concern that beer had seemed to raise blood glucose in the past. Still haven't tried a glass of wine yet.

2) Starches were of real concern at the beginning. As was mentioned earlier, the Thanksgiving meal at a local restaurant offered only white potatoes or sweet potatoes or yams covered in brown sugar or maple syrup, but they did accommodate my dietary needs by serving pasta and unsweetened sweet potatoes or yams. Two local eateries offer only sandwiches and those sandwiches are only

served on white bread. When I was with my son recently as he picked up a sandwich from one of those cafés, I mentioned the problem with the white bread. I was told to just bring my own bread and they would put the filling on that bread. That is what I did a few days later and the sandwich was both nutritious and delicious.

3) Portion control is always on my mind. Knowing how careful I am at home helps me to relax a little when I am eating out. By that, I do not mean that I give myself permission to eat with abandon. What I mean is that I know I am fairly good at eyeballing portions. When in doubt, I err on the small portion side.

4) There is no Benecol® Light or Light Mayonnaise in restaurants. If I have a salad, I ask for olive oil and vinegar. In restaurants, the danger of consuming too much fat lies in being tempted by things like French fries, but they have been out of my diet since day one of this journey—apart from the Irish fries consumed occasionally. No fried food comes out of my kitchen anymore. Anything cooked in a frying pan is sautéed in olive or cooked in a pan sprayed with non-stick cooking spray.

That's about it for eating out and fast food. Most of the time, I eat at home. With that in mind, I have included some of my favorite easy recipes in Chapter 24. Like everything else that I do to keep the blood glucose under control, I like to KEEP IT SIMPLE.

Part VIII

Shopping and Cooking

SHOPPING LIST/SERVING SIZES

More die in the United States of too much food
than of too little.
JOHN KENNETH GALBRAITH

The modified diet now consists of approximately 1400-1500 calories, made up as follows:

5 servings of starches
3 servings of non-starchy vegetables
2 servings of fruit
2 servings of milk
6 servings of protein
3-4 servings of fat
1 serving of alcohol

STARCHES: (each serving should equal approximately 15 grams of carbohydrate)

Bread: Buns (whole wheat)
Pumpernickel
Rye
Sprouted Barley
Sprouted Rye Seed

Bread (continued)
　　Sprouted Sourdough
　　Sprouted Wheat
　　Stoneground Whole Wheat
Buckwheat Groats
Buckwheat Pancakes
Bulgur Wheat
Couscous
Crackers (whole wheat)
English Muffins (whole wheat)
Flour (stoneground whole wheat)
Kasha
Oatmeal (steelcut)
Pasta (whole wheat preferred)
Pita (whole wheat)
Rice (brown Basmati)
Taco Shells

STARCHY VEGETABLES: (each serving should equal 1/2 cup cooked or 3 ounces uncooked)

Peas (green)
Sweet Potatoes or Yams

STARCH/PROTEIN: (each serving should equal 1/2 cup cooked and is counted as both a starch and a protein serving)

Garbanzo Beans
Kidney Beans
Lentils
Pinto Beans
Split Peas
White Beans

NON-STARCHY VEGETABLES: (each serving should equal 1/2 cup cooked or 1 cup raw)

Asparagus
Beans

Bean Sprouts
Broccoli
Brussels Sprouts
Cabbage
Cauliflower
Celery
Cucumber
Eggplant
Leeks
Mushrooms
Onions (yellow and red)
Pea Pods
Peppers (green, red, yellow)
Salad Greens:
    Chicory
    Endive
    Escarole
    Lettuce:
        Boston Bib
        Iceberg
        Romaine
Scallions
Spinach (fresh and frozen)
Sugar Snap Peas
Tomatoes (canned and fresh)

FRUIT/FRUIT JUICE: (each serving should equal 1/2 cup juice or approximately 4 ounces of fruit)

Apples
Applesauce (unsweetened)
Apricots
Blackberries
Blueberries
Cantaloupe Melon
Cherries
Grapefruit
Grapes
Honeydew Melon

Oranges
Papaya
Peaches
Pears
Plums
Raspberries
Strawberries

Grapefruit Juice (fresh-squeezed)
Orange Juice (fresh-squeezed)

MILK: (each serving should equal 1 cup milk or 2/3 cup yogurt)

Buttermilk
Low-Fat Yogurt
Milk (1% preferred)

PROTEIN: (each serving should equal 1 ounce of cheese, fish, meat, or poultry, 3 slices of bacon, 1 tablespoon of peanut butter, 1 egg, 2 ounces of ricotta cheese, 1/4 cup low-fat cottage cheese, 2 tablespoons of grated parmesan cheese, 1 ounce turkey sausage, 2 sardines, 2 ounces of tofu or 2 anchovies)

Cheese:
Cheddar (50% fat-free preferred)
Cottage Cheese (low-fat)
Mozzarella
Parmesan (grated)
Ricotta
Swiss

Eggs (brown corn-fed)

Fish:
Flounder or other flat fish
Salmon (fresh, canned, or Lox)
Sardines
Swordfish
Tuna (canned)

Meat:
    Beef:
        Corned
        Ground
        Steak
        Stewing Meat
    Lamb:
        Chops
        Ground
        Leg of
        Stewing Meat
    Pork:
        Bacon
        Ham
        Tenderloin

Peanut Butter

Poultry:
    Chicken:
        Breasts
        Cold-Cuts
        Whole
    Turkey:
        Cold-Cuts
        Sausage
        Whole

Shellfish:
    Lobster
    Shrimp

Tofu

FATS: (each serving equals 1 tablespoon of Benecol® Light or light mayonnaise, 1 teaspoon of olive oil, 1 ounce of avocado, or 2 tablespoons of sour cream)

    Avocado
    Benecol® Light
    Light Mayonnaise

Olive Oil
Sour Cream

ALCOHOL:

5 ounces of wine
12 ounce beer
1 1/2 ounces of distilled spirits

MISCELLANEOUS:

Anchovies (sparingly)	Free
Bouillon (beef or chicken)	Free
Capers	Free
Chicken Broth	Free
Chives	Free
Coffee	Free
Cooking Spray (no-stick)	Free
Garlic	Free
Herbs and Spices	Free
Lemon Juice	Free
Lime Juice	Free
Mustard	Free
Pepper	Free
Salt	Free
Soy Sauce	Free
Spaghetti Sauce	(count the carbs)
Tabasco	Free
Taco Sauce	Free
Tea	Free
Tomato Paste	Free
Vinegar (balsamic, wine and white)	Free
Wine (red and white cooking)	Free
Worcestershire Sauce	Free

~ **23** ~

PRODUCT PREFERENCES

Let us prefer, let us not exclude.

JOSEPH ROUX

STARCHES

Bread:

Pumpernickel	Pepperidge Farm® Dark
Rye	Pepperidge Farm®
Sprouted Barley	Alvarado Street Bakery®
Sprouted Rye Seed	Alvarado Street Bakery®
Sprouted Sourdough	Alvarado Street Bakery®
Sprouted Wheat	Alvarado Street Bakery®
Stoneground Whole Wheat	Wonder® 100%
Buckwheat Groats	Wolff's® Whole
Buckwheat Pancakes	Arrowhead Mills® Buckwheat Pancake & Waffle Mix
Crackers	Wasa® Crispbread Multi-Grain
Couscous	Rice Select™ Whole Wheat
English Muffins	Thomas'® Hearty Grains
Oatmeal	John McCann's(U) Steelcut
Pasta (whole wheat)	Hodson Mill® Angel Hair
	Hodgson Mill® Fettuccini
	Hodgson Mill® Spaghetti
	Ronzoni™ Healthy Harvest Pasta
	Ronzoni™ Healthy Harvest Penne

	Ronzoni™ Healthy Harvest Rotini
Pita	Thomas'® Sahara Whole Wheat Pita
Rice	Della® Gourmet Rice Aromatic American Basmati Brown Rice
Taco Shells	Old El Paso®

NON-STARCHY VEGETABLES

Beans (green, frozen)	Hanover® Petite
Brussels Sprouts (frozen)	Hanover® Petite
Sugar Snap Peas (frozen)	Hanover® Petite

MILK

Low-Fat Yogurt	Stoneyfield Farms®

PROTEIN

Bacon	Try Oscar's English, Irish, or Canadian (Call 1-800-627-3431)
Cheese (cheddar)	Cabot's® 50% Light Vermont
Peanut Butter	Smucker's® Creamy
Sausage	Armor® Brown'N Serve Fully Cooked Turkey Sausage Links

FATS

Mayonnaise	Hellman's® Light
Spread	Benecol® Light

MISCELLANEOUS

Cooking Spray (no-stick)	Pam® 100% Extra Virgin Olive Oil Pam® Butter Flavor

~ 24 ~

RECIPES

The discovery of a new dish does more for human happiness than the discovery of a star.
ANTHELME BRILLAT-SAVARIN

NOTES ON THE FOLLOWING RECIPES

❑ <u>Starches:</u> All lunch and dinner meals provide two starch servings. The one breakfast meal provides one starch serving.

❑ <u>Protein:</u> Most meals provide two protein servings for lunch and three protein servings for dinner. Sometimes, it is difficult to modify the recipe to reduce from three protein servings to two protein servings. If a meal with three protein servings is served at lunch, it is easy to reduce the dinner meal to include only two portions of protein. One recipe provides 2 1/2 protein servings per meal. Again, it is easy to adjust the other meal of the day or to enjoy the same meal twice in the same day. The breakfast recipe provides just one protein serving.

❑ <u>Fruit:</u> Fruit is usually reserved for 4 ounces of juice with dinner and 4 ounces of fruit in the afternoon. Occasionally fruit is added in small measure to the recipes—two ounces of apple sauce with roast pork or 1/2 ounce of blueberries in the buckwheat pancakes. This just calls for reducing the afternoon fruit by the amount consumed earlier, or to be consumed later, in the day.

❑ <u>Vegetables:</u> Vegetables are not measured precisely. Some recipes provide 1 1/2 servings of vegetables for lunch and for dinner per meal. If the amount included in a recipe is less than the 1 1/2 servings allowed per meal, a small salad might be added or vegetables might be increased at the other meal of the day. When a salad is served, this is always dressed with olive oil and balsamic vinegar.

❑ <u>Fat:</u> Fat is sometimes measured, sometimes not. It is my practice to go sparingly with the Benecol® Light, the Hellman's® Light Mayonnaise, the olive oil, and the sour cream. A small slice of avocado is used occasionally. Nothing in these recipes is deep-fried. Some recipes call for stir-frying vegetables with olive oil. Often, no-stick cooking sprays are used.

❑ <u>Milk:</u> If milk is included in the recipe, it is easy to reduce the milk for the rest of the day.

❑ <u>Salt:</u> Salt is added to recipes very sparingly and only if the recipe is being shared with others.

❑ <u>Wine:</u> Wine is optional in two recipes. In neither of these recipes does the wine amount to much more than one ounce per meal.

ONE LAST WORD ON CARBOHYDRATES

It is easiest for me to think in terms of carbohydrates as five starches, two glasses of milk, and two fruits per day. Once in a while, a recipe calls for something like spaghetti sauce which adds a small amount of carbohydrate to the recipe. An adjustment is made for this by reducing the rest of the starch amount per meal. Stoneground whole wheat flour is called for in a few recipes. The amount in each meal is rather insignificant and is not included in the carbohydrate totals.

FISH

Poached Salmon with Mayonnaise Sauce
Salmon with Basmati Rice, Garlic, Onions & Mushrooms
Swordfish Kabobs

BEEF

Beef Burgundy
Tacos
Beef Stroganoff

LAMB

Roast Leg of Lamb with Mint Sauce & Roasted Sweet Potatoes or
Yams
Shepherd's Pie
Lamb Stew with Sweet Potatoes or Yams

PORK

Roast Pork Tenderloin
Pork & Bulgur Casserole
Blueberry Buckwheat Pancakes & Bacon

POULTRY

Cavatelli, Chicken & Broccoli
Turkey Breast with Tuna & Anchovy Sauce
Chicken Noodle Soup

EGGS/CHEESE

Basmati Rice Crust Quiche
Lasagna
Whole Wheat Rotini, Cheese & Spinach Bake

POACHED SALMON WITH MAYONNAISE SAUCE

Ingredients:
- 4 ounces low-fat mayonnaise
- 1 small onion, cut into 4 pieces
- Several leaves fresh parsley, chopped coarsely
- 1 tablespoon white vinegar
- l pound salmon (trimmed of skin & dark middle yields about 12 ounces)
- 8 servings couscous for dinner, 3/4 cup uncooked (12 servings for lunch, 1 cup uncooked)

Cooking Instructions:
- In a blender, blend together mayonnaise, onion, parsley, & vinegar & refrigerate
- Cut salmon into 4 portions for dinner (6 portions for lunch)
- Poach or steam salmon until center is cooked
- While salmon is cooking, prepare couscous according to package directions
- Serve salmon with warm couscous
- Drizzle salmon with mayonnaise sauce

MEALS
Dinner (4)
Lunch (6)

COMPLETE THE MEAL
Add vegetables or a salad.

SUGGESTIONS
Cook more salmon than needed and use for the Salmon with Basmati Rice, Garlic, Onions & Mushrooms recipe.

SALMON WITH BASMATI RICE, GARLIC, ONIONS & MUSHROOMS

Ingredients:
- 1 pound salmon (trimmed of skin & dark middle yields about 12 ounces)
- 2 tablespoons olive oil
- Several cloves garlic, chopped
- 2 cups onions, chopped
- 2 cups mushrooms, chopped
- 8 servings cooked Basmati rice for dinner, 7/8th cup uncooked (12 servings cooked for lunch, 1 1/4 cup uncooked)
- Salt, to taste

Cooking Instructions:
- Cut salmon into 4 portions for dinner (6 for lunch)
- Poach or steam salmon until center is cooked
- Crumble cooked salmon into bit-sized pieces
- Heat olive oil in large frying pan
- Stir-fry garlic, onions & mushrooms until lightly browned
- Add cooked Basmati rice & continue to stir-fry until warm
- Remove from heat & mix in crumbled salmon
- Salt, to taste

MEALS
Dinner (4)
Lunch (6)

COMPLETE THE MEAL
Add vegetables or a salad.

SWORDFISH KABOBS

Ingredients:
- 1 pound swordfish (trimmed of skin & dark middle yields about 12 ounces)
- 4 small onions for dinner (6 for lunch)
- 8 small mushrooms for dinner (12 for lunch)
- 1 large tomato cut into 8 pieces for dinner (1 1/2 cut into 12 pieces for lunch)
- 1/2 green pepper cut into 8 pieces for dinner (3/4 cut into 12 for lunch)
- 2 lemons
- No-stick olive oil cooking spray
- Salt & pepper, to taste
- 8 servings couscous for dinner, 3/4 cup uncooked (12 servings for lunch, 1 cup uncooked)

Cooking Instructions:
- Heat broiler on hi setting
- Cut swordfish into 20 small pieces for dinner (30 for lunch)
- Prepare vegetables by peeling onions & washing mushrooms
- Place ingredients on 4 skewers for dinner (6 for lunch) in the following order: onion, fish, mushroom, fish, tomato, pepper, fish, pepper, fish, tomato, fish, mushroom
- Spray broiler pan with no-stick olive oil cooking spray
- Place Kabobs on broiler pan
- Squeeze juice of lemons & spray no-stick olive oil cooking spray over all sides of Kabobs
- Season with salt & pepper, to taste
- Grill for three minutes, turn & grill for three more minutes, turn again & grill for 3 more minutes
- While Kabobs are cooking, prepare couscous according to package directions
- Serve Kabobs over couscous

MEALS
Dinner (4)
Lunch (6)

BEEF BURGUNDY

Ingredients:
- 3 tablespoons olive oil, divided
- 9 pieces Canadian bacon, cut into bite sized pieces
- 1 cup onions, sliced
- 1 1/4 pounds beef stew, cut into one inch squares
- 1/4 cup stoneground whole wheat flour
- 1 beef bouillon cube dissolved in 3 cups hot water
- 1 cup mushrooms, sliced
- 2 dried bay leaves
- 2 tablespoons fresh parsley, chopped
- 1 teaspoon dried thyme
- Salt, to taste
- 1 cup red wine, optional

Cooking Instructions:
- Pre-heat oven to 350°
- Heat 2 tablespoons olive oil in large frying pan & brown bacon & onions
- When browned, spoon bacon & onions into large oven-proof casserole dish
- Add another tablespoon of olive oil to frying pan
- Add meat to pan turning often until well browned on all sides
- Sprinkle flour over meat & blend with wooden spoon
- Pour hot water & bouillon over meat & bring to a boil
- Transfer meat mixture to casserole dish
- Add mushrooms, herbs, & salt to taste
- Add red wine
- Stir pot
- Cover with lid & cook in pre-heated oven for 4 hours

MEALS
Dinner (6)
Lunch (9)

<u>Complete the Meal</u>
Add vegetables or a salad.
Serve with 2 servings of crusty coarse whole grain bread for each meal.

TACOS

Ingredients:
- 12 ounces ground beef
- Worcestershire sauce, to taste
- Taco sauce, to taste
- Salt & pepper, to taste
- Several leaves romaine lettuce, shredded
- 1 large red onion, chopped
- 1 large ripe tomato, chopped
- Olive oil
- Balsamic vinegar
- 16 crispy taco shells for dinner (24 for lunch)
- 3 ounces cheddar cheese, grated
- Sour cream

Cooking Instructions:
- Pre-heat oven to 250°
- Fry meat in non-stick frying pan until well-browned
- Add Worcestershire sauce, taco sauce, & salt & pepper, to taste
- In medium-sized bowl mix together lettuce, onion, & tomato
- Toss salad with olive oil, balsamic vinegar, & salt & pepper, to taste
- Put tacos on metal cookie sheet & warm in pre-heated oven for about 4 minutes
- When tacos are warm, spread the meat mixture between them & then add the vegetables on top
- Finish with the shredded cheese & a small dollop of sour cream

MEALS
Dinner (4)
Lunch (6)

BEEF STROGANOFF

Ingredients:
- 1 pound ground beef
- 1 large onion, chopped
- 2 cloves garlic, minced
- 8 ounces fresh mushrooms, chopped
- 1 beef bouillon dissolved in 1 cup hot water
- 1 tablespoon tomato paste
- 1/2 cup sour cream
- 1 tablespoon stoneground whole wheat flour
- Salt & pepper, to taste
- 8 servings whole wheat noodles for dinner, 6 ounces uncooked (12 servings for lunch, 9 ounces uncooked)

Cooking Instructions:
- Fry meat in non-stick frying pan until well-browned
- Add onion, garlic, & mushrooms
- Continue to saute until onion is lightly browned
- Pour meat & vegetables into crock-pot
- Add bouillon & tomato paste to crock-pot stirring until well mixed
- Cover & cook on low for 8-10 hours
- 30 minutes before serving, stir in sour cream & flour
- Just before serving, add salt & pepper, to taste
- Cook noodles according to package directions
- Serve contents of crock-pot over hot noodles

MEALS
Dinner (4)
Lunch (6)

COMPLETE THE MEAL
Add vegetables or a salad.

ROAST LEG OF LAMB WITH MINT SAUCE & ROASTED SWEET POTATOES OR YAMS

Ingredients:
- Leg of lamb
- Several cloves of garlic, sliced into long pieces
- Stoneground whole wheat flour for dredging
- Large bunch of fresh mint, chopped finely
- 1/2 cup red wine vinegar
- 1 1/2 pounds sweet potatoes or yams, peeled & cut into large roasting size pieces
- Benecol® Light

Cooking Instructions:
- Preheat oven to 350°
- Rinse leg of lamb & place in roasting pan
- Cut slits in fat deposits on lamb & insert slices of garlic
- Sprinkle flour over lamb
- Place roasting pan in pre-heated oven & cook for 45 minutes per pound or until meat thermometer registers 180°
- Mix mint with red wine vinegar, refrigerate
- 1 1/2 hours before lamb is expected to be done, par-boil sweet potatoes or yams for about 10 minutes
- Melt enough Benecol® Light in a separate roasting pan to roast potatoes
- Put par-boiled potatoes in hot Benecol® Light & turn often to brown potatoes
- Serve lamb (3 ounces per meal for dinner; 2 ounces per meal for lunch) with mint sauce sprinkled over the top & roasted potatoes on the side

MEALS
Dinner (4)
Lunch (4)

COMPLETE THE MEAL
Add vegetables or a salad.

Suggestion

Mince enough meat for Shepherd's Pie recipe. Use left over meat for sandwiches.

SHEPHERD'S PIE

Ingredients:
- 2 1/4 pounds sweet potatoes or yams, peeled & cut into small cubes
- 6 tablespoons Benecol® Light, divided
- 2 medium onions, chopped
- 18 ounces minced cooked lamb for dinner (12 ounces for lunch)
- 3 tablespoons stoneground whole wheat flour
- 1 bouillon cube dissolved in 1 cup hot water
- Salt & pepper, to taste
- 4 ounces of 1% milk

Cooking Instructions:
- Pre-heat oven to 425°
- Put the potatoes on to boil
- Melt one tablespoon of Benecol® Light in medium frying pan & brown the onion
- Stir in minced lamb
- Add the flour & cook for 2-3 minutes
- Add dissolved bouillon & stir until boiling
- Boil gently for five minutes.
- Season with salt & pepper, to taste
- Drain & mash the potatoes
- Beat 5 tablespoons of Benecol® Light & the milk into the potatoes
- Season potatoes with salt & pepper, to taste
- Spread meat in bottom of oven-proof dish and top with mashed potatoes
- Cook in preheated oven for about 30 minutes & finish with a quick browning under the grill

MEALS
Dinner (6)
Lunch (6)

COMPLETE THE MEAL
Add vegetables or a salad.

LAMB STEW WITH SWEET POTATOES OR YAMS

Ingredients:
- 1 beef bouillon dissolved in 1 cup hot water
- 1 1/2 pounds lamb stew meat, cut into bite-sized pieces for dinner (1 pound for lunch)
- 2 onions, chopped
- 1 stalk celery, chopped
- 1/2 teaspoon dried marjoram
- 1/2 teaspoon dried thyme
- Salt & pepper, to taste
- 2 1/4 pounds sweet potatoes, peeled & cut into bite-sized pieces
- 3 tablespoons stoneground whole wheat flour
- 1/4 cup water
- 2 cups frozen peas

Cooking Instructions:
- Combine dissolved bouillon, meat, onions, celery, herbs & salt & pepper to taste in crock-pot
- Cover & cook on low for 8-10 hours
- Add sweet potatoes during last 2 hours of cooking
- Dissolve flour in water & stir into stew
- Turn heat up to high & cover & cook for an additional 20 minutes
- Add peas during last 10 minutes of cooking

MEALS
Dinner (6)
Lunch (6)

COMPLETE THE MEAL
Add a small salad.

ROAST PORK TENDERLOIN

Ingredients:
- Pork tenderloin between 2 to 3 pounds
- 12 servings whole wheat noodles, 9 ounces uncooked
- Benecol® Light
- 6 ounces unsweetened apple sauce

Cooking Instructions:
- Pre-heat oven to 350°
- Place tenderloin on a rack over drip pan
- Cook in preheated oven for about 30 minutes per pound or until a meat thermometer registers at least 185°
- Cook noodles according to package instructions & toss with Benecol® Light
- Serve pork with apple sauce & hot noodles

MEALS
Dinner (6) (serve 3 ounces cooked meat per meal)
Lunch (6) (serve 2 ounces cooked meat per meal)

COMPLETE THE MEAL
Add vegetables or a salad.

SUGGESTION
Use left-over pork to make delicious sandwiches on whole wheat bread spread with light mayonnaise and finished with lettuce & tomato slices or use in the Pork & Bulgur Casserole recipe.

PORK & BULGUR CASSEROLE

Ingredients:
- 8 ounces cooked pork, cubed
- 28 ounce tin whole tomatoes with juice
- 2 onions, chopped
- 8 ounces mushrooms, chopped
- 8 servings bulgur for dinner, 3/4 cup uncooked (12 servings for lunch, 1 cup uncooked)
- Salt & pepper, to taste
- 4 ounces shredded Swiss cheese

Cooking Instructions:
- Pre-heat oven to 375°
- Mix pork, tomatoes, onions, mushrooms, bulgur, & salt & pepper, to taste
- Cover & cook for 45 minutes
- Uncover & spread shredded cheese on top
- Place under grill until browned

MEALS
Dinner (4)
Lunch (6)

COMPLETE THE MEAL
Add vegetables or a salad.

BLUEBERRY BUCKWHEAT PANCAKES & BACON

Ingredients:
- 12 slices lean bacon
- 2/3 cup Arrowhead Mills® Buckwheat Pancake & Waffle Mix
- Water to mix
- No-stick butter cooking spray
- 2 ounces blueberries, washed & dried
- Benecol® Light

Cooking Instructions:
- Fry bacon, drain on paper towels
- Mix pancake mix with water only to form a fairly thick batter
- Heat large non-stick frying pan & spray with no-stick butter cooking spray
- When pan is heated, add buckwheat pancake mixture to form 4 pancakes
- Brown on one side
- Drop blueberries in equal numbers on the uncooked surface of the 4 pancakes
- Turn
- When brown on both sides, serve on 4 plates
- Spread each pancake with Benecol® Light
- Add 3 slices bacon to each plate

MEALS
Breakfast (4)

COMPLETE THE MEAL
1/2 glass of milk per meal rounds out this "once-in-a-while" breakfast treat.

SUGGESTION
Breakfast is a meal that we often make just for ourselves, and it is nice to be able to adapt a recipe to serve one person. It is difficult to measure 1/6th of a cup of dry mix in a one cup measure to make one buckwheat pancake, but here's a way to solve that problem.

Using a four-ounce measuring glass, pour in just less than three tablespoons of dry pancake mix. To this, add water and stir with a teaspoon until the desired consistency is obtained. Continue with the recipe, but add just 1/2 ounce blueberries and serve with three slices of bacon.

CAVATELLI, CHICKEN & BROCOLLI

Ingredients:
- 5 frozen 4 ounce chicken breasts for dinner (3 for lunch)
- 16 ounces frozen cavatelli
- 3 heads broccoli, washed & cut into small florets
- 3 tablespoons olive oil
- Several cloves of garlic, chopped
- 5 ounces cheddar cheese for dinner, grated (4 ounces for lunch)
- 1 ounce Parmesan cheese

Cooking Instructions:
- Cook frozen chicken breasts in oven according to package directions
- When chicken breasts are cooked, set oven temperature to 350°
- Cook cavatelli according to package directions
- For last 6 minutes of cooking time, add broccoli florets to the boiling water, drain
- Cut chicken breasts into bite-sized pieces
- In frying pan, heat olive oil & lightly brown garlic
- In large baking dish pour in cavatelli & broccoli, mix in chicken pieces, pour in olive oil & garlic, mix in grated cheddar cheese, top with grated parmesan
- Put baking dish in pre-heated oven & cook for 40 minutes

MEALS
Lunch (7)
Dinner (7)

COMPLETE THE MEAL
Add a small salad.

TURKEY BREAST WITH TUNA & ANCHOVY SAUCE

Ingredients:
- 1/2 cup low-fat mayonnaise
- 6 ounce tin tuna packed in water
- 6 anchovies
- Small onion, cut into 4 pieces
- 8 capers
- 2 thick slices turkey, each slice weighing about 6 ounces
- 6 ounces whole wheat noodles cooked according to package directions for dinner (9 ounces for lunch)
- Benecol® Light

Cooking Instructions:
- Put mayonnaise, tuna, anchovies, onion & capers in blender
- Blend all ingredients until smooth then refrigerate until ready for use
- Cut turkey into 4 portions for dinner (6 for lunch)
- Toss cooked noodles with Benecol® Light
- Spread tuna & anchovy sauce over turkey & serve with hot noodles

MEALS
Dinner (4)
Lunch (6)

COMPLETE THE MEAL
Add vegetables or a salad.

CHICKEN NOODLE SOUP

Ingredients:
- 3 onions, sliced
- 3 stalks celery, cut into 3/4 inch pieces
- 3 pound broiler or fryer chicken, rinsed
- 1 teaspoon basil
- Salt & pepper, to taste
- 4 cups water, chicken broth, or white wine
- 6 ounces of whole wheat noodles

Cooking Instructions:
- Place onions & celery in bottom of large crock-pot
- Add chicken
- Sprinkle with basil, & salt & pepper, to taste
- Pour liquid over top of other ingredients
- Cover & cook on low for 8-10 hours
- Remove chicken from crock-pot
- Leave crock-pot on low
- Remove skin & bones from chicken & cut meat into bite-sized pieces
- Add back to the crock-pot 12 ounces of chicken for dinner (8 ounces for lunch)
- Add noodles & cook for another 10 minutes or until noodles are tender

MEALS
Lunch (4)
Dinner (4)

COMPLETE THE MEAL
Add vegetables or a salad.

BASMATI RICE CRUST QUICHE

Ingredients:
- No-stick butter cooking spray
- 8 servings cooked Basmati rice, 7/8 cup uncooked
- 6 slices bacon, fried, drained & crumbled
- 5 ounces Swiss cheese, cut into 1/2" cubes
- 2 cups whole milk
- 3 eggs, lightly beaten
- 1/4 teaspoon nutmeg
- Salt & white pepper, to taste

Cooking Instructions:
- Pre-heat oven to 350°
- Spray a 10" pie plate with no-stick butter cooking spray
- Spread the cooked rice in the pie plate pressing into bottom & up sides. Spread bacon & cheese in bottom of prepared pie plate
- Scald milk in small pan & allow to cool
- Stir beaten eggs, nutmeg, & salt & pepper into milk & pour into pie crust
- Place quiche on baking sheet
- Cook in pre-heated oven for 45 minutes or until tooth-pick inserted into center of quiche comes out clean

MEALS
Dinner (4)
Lunch (4)

COMPLETE THE MEAL
Add vegetables or salad.

SUGGESTION
Reduce milk by 1/2 serving for the day. Each meal provides 2 1/2 servings of protein. Just make the other meal of the day another 2 1/2 protein servings meal—maybe serve the quiche for both meals.

LASAGNA

Ingredients:
- 16 ounces ground beef
- Salt & pepper, to taste
- 28 ounce jar spaghetti sauce
- 16 strips lasagna noodles (14 ounces)
- 1 1/2 pounds ricotta cheese
- 5 ounces mozzarella cheese, shredded
- 4 ounces parmesan cheese, divided into two
- 3 eggs, lightly beaten
- 2 tablespoons parsley, chopped

Cooking Instructions:
- Pre-heat oven to 350 degrees
- Brown meat in non-stick frying pan
- When meat is brown, salt & pepper to taste
- Pour in spaghetti sauce over meat & leave on low
- Cook noodles according to package directions
- While noodles are cooking, mix cheeses (reserve 2 ounces of parmesan cheese), eggs & parsley in medium sized bowl
- Layer ingredients in 13 x 9 inch pan in the following order:
  1/2 cup sauce
  4 noodle strips
  1/3 cheese mixture
  3/4 cup sauce
  4 noodle strips
  1/3 cheese mixture
  3/4 cup sauce
  4 noodle strips
  1/3 cheese mixture
  3/4 cup sauce
  4 noodle strips
  Spread remaining sauce on top
  Sprinkle with remaining 2 ounces parmesan cheese
- Cover with aluminum foil
- Cook in pre-heated for 30 minutes
- Remove foil & cook for 15 minutes longer
- Remove from oven & allow to cool before serving

MEALS
Dinner (12)
Lunch (not adaptable to lunch). If lasagna is consumed at lunch-time, simply use a meal with only two protein servings for dinner.

COMPLETE THE MEAL
Add vegetables or a salad.

WHOLE WHEAT ROTINI, CHEESE & SPINACH BAKE

Ingredients:
- No-stick butter cooking spray
- 2 eggs, lightly beaten
- 1/2 cup ricotta cheese
- 4 ounces mozzarella cheese for dinner, grated (2 ounces for lunch)
- 1 package frozen chopped spinach cooked according to package directions and drained
- 2 1/4 cups whole wheat rotini cooked according to package directions and drained
- Salt & pepper, to taste
- 4 ounces cheddar cheese for dinner, grated (2 ounces for lunch)

Cooking Instructions:
- Pre-heat oven to 375°
- Spray an 8-inch square baking pan with no-stick butter cooking spray
- Mix together eggs, ricotta cheese, mozzarella cheese, spinach and rotini in large bowl
- Salt & pepper, to taste
- Spoon into prepared baking pan
- Cover with cheddar cheese
- Cook in pre-heated oven uncovered for 15 minutes, or until lightly browned

MEALS
Lunch (4)
Dinner (4)

COMPLETE THE MEAL
Add vegetables or salad.

Afterword

Hemoglobin A1c and Lipid Panel results from 4/10/2006 compared with earlier results:

	4/10/06	10/13/05	3/28/05	3/18/05
Hemoglobin A1c				
Hemoglobin A1c	5.7	5.7	12.9	
Mean Blood Glucose	114.6	114.6	342.8	
Glucose				389
Lipid Panel				
Cholesterol	186	191		302
Triglycerides	76	88		282
HDL	65	52		30
vLDL	15.2	17.6		56.4
cLDL	105.8	121.4		215.6
Chol/HDL Ratio	2.9	3.7		10.1
LDL/HDL Ratio	1.6	2.3		7.2